The Green Bookshop

The Green Bookshop

RECOMMENDED READING FOR DOCTORS
AND OTHERS FROM THE MEDICAL JOURNAL
EDUCATION FOR PRIMARY CARE

JOHN SALINSKY
BM BCh MRCP FRCGP
General Practitioner (London)
Programme Director,
Whittington GP Specialty Training Scheme,
London

with

IONA HEATH
MB BChir MRCGP
General Practitioner
Caversham Group Practice, North London

and

MARY SALINSKY
MA MSc

Radcliffe Publishing
Oxford • New York

Radcliffe Publishing Ltd
18 Marcham Road
Abingdon
Oxon OX14 1AA
United Kingdom

www.radcliffe-oxford.com
Electronic catalogue and worldwide online ordering facility.

British Library Cataloguing in Publication Data

A catalogue record for this book is available from the British Library.

ISBN-13: 978 184619 330 9

Typeset by Pindar NZ, Auckland, New Zealand
Printed and bound by Cadmus Communications, USA

Contents

Preface

What makes a perfect bookshop? For me the London Review of Books Bookshop in London comes very close. It is not very big but the books are chosen with such care that the choice is always both intriguing and beguiling and it is very rare for me to summon the restraint necessary to leave empty-handed. It also includes a delightful little café with very good coffee and cakes that are much too tempting. John Salinsky's Green Bookshop has all these components, with a particular emphasis on the importance of the coffee, but it is even better on two counts: firstly, his selection is equally broad but it has a subtle slant informed by his years of listening and talking to patients in general practice; and then there is the gentle erudition and commitment of the proprietor himself.

John believes in books as a force for good in the world in general and within general practice in particular. He relishes the power of words to help us make sense of what happens in the worlds around and within us and perhaps particularly to help us to understand the predicament of the other, of those whose experience of life is so different from our own. He believes in the capacity of books to enlarge our sympathies, our outlook and our experience and he knows that this potential is particularly important for doctors. He offers his own delight in books and sets out to tempt his customers to open a book and begin reading but he is never didactic, never seeks to impose his own view or interpretation. His hope is to share one of the great pleasures of his life.

John carefully mines books for 'beautiful insights' and 'little images' which stay with him and change his view of the world and of the struggles of his patients within it. He is intrigued by the presence of doctors both as writers and as characters and much of his belief in the importance of literature for doctors is captured in the quotation he selects from Ian McEwan's *Atonement*:

> For this was the point, surely: he would be a better doctor for having read literature. What deep readings his modified sensibility might make of human suffering, of the self-destructive folly or sheer bad luck that drives men towards ill health! Birth, death and frailty in between. Rise and fall – this was the doctor's business and it was literature's, too.

I envy John his hours spent in the peace and comfort of this marvellous bookshop, waiting for customers and reading, always reading. I want to read or re-read every book that he mentions and somehow I must find the time to do this. One obvious and very attractive solution would be to give up paying any attention to the degraded use of words that makes up so much of the policy literature of healthcare and the health service. What a liberation that would be.

On the basis of John Salinsky's first volume on *Medicine and Literature*, I resolved to read *Tristram Shandy* and within its magnificent prodigality I found, among much else, some wonderful ripostes to the contemporary abuse of words:

> – their heads, Sir, are stuck so full of rules and compasses, and have that eternal propensity to apply them upon all occasions, that a work of genius had better go to the devil at once, than stand to be pricked and tortured to death by 'em.

This time, in *The Green Bookshop*, I have found the perfect gift for my husband's next birthday but its identity must remain a secret. Thank you John.

Iona Heath
April 2009

About the authors

John Salinsky is a general practitioner in North West London and a Programme Director at the Whittington GP Specialty Training Scheme. He is the author of *Medicine and Literature, Volumes 1 and 2* (published in 2002 and 2004, respectively, by Radcliffe Publishing). Since 2001, he has written book reviews for the journal *Education for Primary Care* (Radcliffe Publishing) in a regular column entitled 'The Green Bookshop.'

Iona Heath has been an inner-city general practitioner at the Caversham Group Practice in Kentish Town in London since 1975. She has been a nationally elected member of the Council of the Royal College of General Practitioners since 1989, and chaired the College's Committee on Medical Ethics from 1998 to 2004. She is now chairing the College's International Committee. She also chairs the Ethics Committee of the *British Medical Journal* and is a member of the WONCA World Executive. Her book *Matters of Life and Death* was published in 2008 by Radcliffe Publishing.

Mary Salinsky read history at St Anne's College, Oxford. She worked as a civil servant and subsequently as a research officer for the Medical Foundation for Care of Victims of Torture. She is currently writing a PhD thesis on British historiography.

CHAPTER 1

The Green Bookshop opens its doors

Welcome to the Green Bookshop! When I was invited by the editor of *Education for Primary Care* to take over that journal's book reviews, I decided to open a special bookshop for the benefit of readers. Naturally it had to be called the Green Bookshop. It is painted green so that you can easily find it, and it is just a short walk down the High Street.

Now I know that some of you are already regular customers. One or two of you have been visiting us ever since we opened. But for the benefit of newcomers (who are always welcome) I would like to tell you a bit about the sort of bookshop we are.

We are fiercely independent and will never be part of any large organisation. Our stock is quite small and very carefully chosen. Some might say we are idiosyncratic and even eccentric. To those people I would say: who cares? If you want run-of-the-mill textbooks, carelessly written best-sellers and formulaic genre books, there are plenty of places where you can get them. There is only one Green Bookshop.

Now you may have noticed that we have a substantial medical book department. This is for the benefit of our primary healthcare readers, but even if you are not medical, we hope you will find some interesting and easily readable books there. You don't have to go there at all if you don't want to, although you might want to take a look at what your friendly local GP and their colleagues are reading.

So what sort of books do we have for you?

➤ The best novels by living writers, especially those that have won, or nearly won, prizes.

➤ Books which have something new to say about primary care.

➤ Books which might help us doctors to look after our patients better.

➤ Almost anything that is really well written.

➤ Classics, which come up fresh however often you read them.

➤ Some history, some biography, and some books by Deep Thinkers.

➤ *And books featuring feisty women. And books about love.*

Yes indeed. Thank you, Dorothy. Ladies and gentlemen, let me introduce Miss Dorothy Malone, who is my invaluable assistant in the Green Bookshop. Dorothy has many roles, and I don't know how I would manage without her. She presides at the cash desk and knows all about credit cards, she chooses the blends for the coffee machine, and she designs the unique Green Bookshop carrier bags.

And what else do I do? You supply what one might call the woman's angle when we are evaluating the books. The feminine touch without which we would be incomplete. *OK, I guess that will do for now. But let's not forget that some of the best writers in the world have been women, and there would have been more if they had not had to struggle against male oppression with no access to education. Oh yes, and the majority of GPs are now women.* Thank you, Dorothy.

You can see that we love debate and controversy at the Green Bookshop. One of the great pleasures of presiding here is the way people come in for a chat. They ask if we have some book or other, and very often it will be something I know well and have strong views about. Soon we are absorbed in a lively discussion about the book and its author and have you read this and what about that? Other customers come and join in, and it gets very lively indeed, I can tell you.

On the other hand, there are times when business is slow and Dorothy is away, when it gets a bit lonely behind the counter. I sit here (with a book, naturally) and I find myself getting into strange states of altered consciousness. Not due to drugs, I assure you, unless reading is a drug, which it very likely is, come to think of it. Sometimes I imagine I am a character from fiction. Other times the shop door opens in my dreams and in comes Mr Pickwick or someone from Jane Austen.

I don't think it's good for him to be too long here by himself. It brings out his Samuel Beckett tendencies. He ought to get out a bit more and let me be in charge. Dorothy, you are right as usual.

But now I can see a few of you outside the shop, peering through the window at me. Don't be afraid, you will be free to browse undisturbed for as long as you like. You don't have to buy anything. You can even help yourself to a cup of coffee. And every day, at three o'clock, we will give you a special presentation focusing on a different aspect of the literary treasures to be found on our shelves. As you cautiously open the door, a little bell chimes softly. Welcome to the Green Bookshop!

CHAPTER 2

Books that won prizes

Here at the Green Bookshop we are very interested in literary prizes, and especially the most famous one awarded in the UK, the Booker, now known as the Man Booker Prize. These competitions get a lot of publicity in the media, the bookies quote odds on who is going to win, there are interviews with the shortlisted writers, and there is a sort of Oscar-style ceremony when the prize is eventually awarded in October. The winner and everyone on the short list get a big boost in their sales. And then it's all over for another year. But why should we bother to get excited? Well, the fact that a book has got on to the short list usually (although not always) means that it is one of the best of the year and, with all the thousands of books demanding our attention these days, it's not a bad guide to what is worth reading. Some prize winners are really great books, and a few have already become classics (like Salman Rushdie's *Midnight's Children*). On the other hand, there are some terrific books that have not won prizes. So in this chapter we are presenting just a selection of the prize winners of the last seven years – the ones we really think you should read. And in the next chapter we will tell you about some equally good books that should have won prizes, but didn't.

So now, let us start the parade of the prize winners.

The Booker Prize 2001: *TRUE HISTORY OF THE KELLY GANG* by Peter Carey

In case you are not Australian, let me tell you a bit about Ned Kelly. He was a bandit of Irish origin, who flourished in the colony of Victoria in the 1870s and 1880s, and became a folk hero rather like our own Robin Hood.

According to the legend, he and his gang robbed the rich, helped the poor and only shot policemen in self-defence. But what *was* the 'true history' of the Kelly gang? Peter Carey imagined himself into Ned Kelly's mind and created a very effective, slightly ungrammatical but intensely personal literary style for Ned to use in telling his story. We readers are asked to imagine that he wrote his autobiography on any scraps of paper he could get hold of and carefully wrapped them up in 13 parcels, to be read by his daughter after his death. Here is an example in which he talks about his mother:

> One morning in the summer of 1872 my mother were 42 yr old she had 2 sons in prison also 1 brother & 1 uncle & 1 brother in law. 2 of her beloved daughters was buried beneath the willow tree and God knows what worse was on the way.

Ned's mother is very important in his life. After the death of her husband, she does her best to run a poor little farm and bring up her children. But, to her son's disgust, she attracts a succession of undesirable new 'husbands' who climb into her bed, produce more young siblings and then disappear. At the age of 14, Ned finds himself 'apprenticed' to a colourful highwayman called Harry Power who is one of his mother's lovers. Harry teaches him to survive in the bush and involves him in some rather incompetent (and entertaining) attempts at holding up stagecoaches. Soon he is fully launched on a career as a bandit, horse-thief and gunman. As we read, we get to know Ned's younger brothers and sisters and feel almost like one of the family. There are frequent intrusions by policemen, who may appear friendly but are not to be trusted. Constable Fitzpatrick comes courting Ned's sister Kate and receives a blow on the head from Mrs Kelly's shovel. When he draws his gun on her, Ned shoots him in the hand. His mother is arrested and imprisoned, which makes young Ned very angry and determined to get her released. Ned and his brother Dan, together with some of their closest friends, become the Kelly Gang. Three policemen are shot dead when they try to ambush the Kellys. The gang become bank robbers, and seem to be well liked by the local people to whom Ned tries to explain that he would never have become an outlaw if the police had left him and his family in peace. Each stage of his horrendous descent into crime seems unwilling and yet inevitable.

Was Ned Kelly really such a tragic hero? It's impossible to say, and as this is a novel, it doesn't really matter. The narrative is utterly convincing, and you soon get used to the lack of commas. The battles and confrontations are really exciting, and there is also some poetic description, a good deal of humour and some tender feeling in the scenes with Mary Hearn, the only love of Ned's brief life. The story begins and ends with an italicised account (not by Ned) of the final battle between the police and the Kellys. The gang are clad in their legendary homemade armour, which unfortunately fails to protect their legs . . .

The Booker Prize 2004: *THE LINE OF BEAUTY* by Alan Hollinghurst

This is a fine novel that offers many treats. First off, it's very skilfully written with none of that infelicity of style that can so easily bring a grimace of pain to the fastidious features of your Green Bookshop reviewer. The story provides an insider's view of the middle Thatcher years (between the 1983 and 1987 elections), interspersed with some very erotic descriptions of gay sex. The hero is young Nick Guest, aged 24 and recently down from Oxford where he met some very posh friends, including Toby Fedden, the son of one of the newly elected Tory MPs. Nick has been invited to take up semi-permanent residence in the Feddens' Notting Hill mansion, where he admires the family's collection of art and antiques and looks after Toby's younger sister Catherine, who is on lithium. Gerald, the father, is an amiably pompous fellow and Nick gets on well with him and with his wife Rachel. But Nick isn't a Conservative sympathiser, so what is he doing in this Tory household? The answer seems to be that he is dedicating his young life to the pursuit of Beauty. He has two male lovers, a young black man with whom he has his first sexual experience, and then a glamorous young Lebanese millionaire with whom he is supposed to be making a film. Nick also enjoys artistic treasures and the comfort of being adopted by a rich family. The 'line of beauty', a phrase used by William Hogarth to describe the curve characteristic of natural forms, presents itself to Nick in various guises. It can be the curve of his lover Leo's buttocks, or a line of Henry James, or even a line of cocaine, waiting to be sniffed up through a tightly rolled twenty-pound note. Nick's adventures in Tory high society are very entertainingly described. There are a number of great set pieces, including a country fête at which the MP has to ingratiate himself, and a party that includes a personal appearance by the Prime Minister herself. While we readers rub our eyes in astonishment, The Lady obligingly accepts Nick's cocaine-fuelled invitation to dance. However, the 1987 election is followed by deaths from AIDS and a scandal involving Gerald the MP, for which Nick is unfairly blamed, and as a result of which he falls from grace. Perhaps he valued beauty too much and human relationships too little. You must decide for yourselves. Whatever your politics and sexual inclinations, *The Line of Beauty* is a really absorbing read.

The Man Booker Prize 2006: *THE SEA* by John Banville

Does the first sentence of a novel contain its essence and tell you everything you need to know? I think it does sometimes, but you have to finish the book and turn back to the first page to find out. And some books only reveal themselves on a second reading. Now what would make a person want to do that? I'll tell you what happened with me and *The Sea*.

John Banville's win was unexpected and disappointing for many, including me (but I do tend to get too emotionally involved with my personal favourite). I much preferred *Never Let Me Go* by Kazuo Ishiguro (*see* Chapter 4). I did read *The Sea*, but it didn't make much impression, and when I heard the result I tried to remember what it had been about. There's a grumpy but endearing elderly narrator called Max who is still grieving over the death of his wife from cancer. He goes to stay at a little seaside town in Ireland, the scene of childhood holidays. One summer, when he was about 11, he became entranced by a middle-class family called the Graces, who were staying at a posh villa called The Cedars. He fell in love, first with the mother (a voluptuous blonde woman) and then with her daughter, Chloe. Chloe has a twin brother called Myles, who is mute. They are both rather sinister. Mr Grace, who is hairy and masculine, seems to sit and watch Max in a rather mocking way. There is also a mysterious young woman called Rose who appears to be the children's governess. These dream-like memories mingle in Max's mind with more painful ones of his wife's last illness (described unsentimentally, without sparing the reader). The book ends with the recollection of a tragic drowning. Banville's style is poetic and allusive. The Irish diction reminded me of Joyce, an old favourite of mine. But he also reads a bit like Proust, when he uses long winding sentences to recall the details of old sensations and states of mind.

I turned back to page one and read the first sentence: *They departed, the gods, on the day of the strange tide.* I read on and things that had been obscure became suddenly clear. To Max at the age of 11, the Grace family had seemed as powerful and mysterious as classical gods and goddesses. On the day of the drowning, there is indeed a strange tide – the sea comes in much further than usual, almost like a tsunami. After that, Max recalls, *I would not swim, no not ever again.* That tide gets several mentions, but I had forgotten that it's right there in the first sentence, along with the gods. What I'm trying to say is that this book is deep, like the sea, and full of strange creatures. It needs to be taken slowly to be fully appreciated. And maybe, like me, you'll want to read it again.

The Man Booker Prize 2007: *THE GATHERING* by Anne Enright

And here, eager to tell you all about it, is my faithful assistant Dorothy Malone. Did it deserve the prize, Dorothy?

Well, I didn't read all the short list, but I had to read this one because it's written by a feisty Irish girl and she's magic with words. The story is told by Veronica, who is number ten in a family of twelve children. They are gathering (hence the title) in Dublin for the funeral of Veronica's beloved slightly older brother Liam, who has sadly drowned himself by walking into the sea with stones in his pockets. There was always something not right about Liam, says Veronica, and she traces his destruction back to an event that happened when the two of them, aged eight and nine, were sent to stay with their grandparents. Now the grandmother (Ada) had a lover called Lambert Nugent who may have abused Liam, although you can't be entirely sure from Veronica's account. She interleaves her report with a lot of memories of past events, some of which she has imagined because she wasn't there, like the time Grandmother Ada first met both her husband and her lover in a hotel foyer in 1925. *Wait a minute, excuse me interrupting, Dorothy.* That's OK, John. *But how can a narrator who is a fictional character dreamt up by the author start imagining events for herself?* Well, you know, John, writers will do this sort of thing nowadays, and it is a bit naughty of them, but it makes for a delicious uncertainty in the whole thing – now did this happen or did it not? And isn't it all made up anyway? *Carry on, Dorothy.* I will so. I'm getting all Irish here. Well, isn't my surname Malone? Now Veronica's siblings include the obligatory types that are present, she tells us, in all large families:

> There is always a drunk. There is always someone who has been interfered with as a child. There is always a colossal success with several houses in various countries to which no one is ever invited. There is a mysterious sister.

Add to those a mother who is so vague she can't remember her own children's names, and you appreciate why Veronica has a love–hate relationship with them. We also get to see something of Veronica's own little family – her husband Tom and her two rather sweet little girls, Rebecca and Emily. They are very lovingly described, although Emily (mother's rival) is a bit of a cat. To tell the truth, Veronica herself, although mordantly witty and likeable, is also a bit worrying. You are never quite sure what she will do next. One minute she tells us she has had sex with Tom for the last time, the night of Liam's funeral, because she wasn't in the mood and he hurt her. Then she suddenly pops up in a hotel at Gatwick Airport and starts talking about having another baby. *And what about the writing, Dorothy. Is it fun to read?* It is, it is. It can be harrowing and unsparing, especially when dealing with death and corpses and cold unfeeling sex, but Veronica, I mean Anne, is also very funny and she's brilliant at evoking the sounds and smells and touch of things. *So you'd recommend it?* Definitely, John.

The Man Booker Prize 2008: *THE WHITE TIGER* by Aravind Adiga

This won after some serious dispute among the judges. It is Aravind's first novel, and it is a pretty impressive achievement. As it is a severely critical book about India by an Indian writer, it inevitably invites comparison with Salman Rushdie's *Midnight's Children*, the 1981 winner, later voted Book of Bookers, which we will discuss a little later (in Chapter 5).

The hero of *The White Tiger* is Balram, a poor boy who has made good by doing some very bad things. He tells his story in the form of a series of memoirs to the premier of China who is about to visit his home town of Bangalore. He will want to meet some of India's new entrepreneurs (known as White Tigers), and Balram promises to tell him the truth. The truth is that Indian society, despite its much praised democracy, is grossly unequal. The rich live in the Light while the poor, like Balram's family, inhabit the Darkness from which it is almost impossible to emerge. Their lives are ruled by corrupt, vicious local landlords who keep their power by bribing the police and the politicians. The millions of poor people have little food, no healthcare and no prospects. They emerge from their partial education as 'half-baked men.' The best a poor man can hope for is to be a rich man's servant.

But Balram has escaped, because he tells us he is now a White Tiger. He also reveals at the end of the first chapter (so I'm not giving much away) that eight months previously he slit the throat of his employer. Naturally, we want to know how and why he did this, and to follow his progress from being the degraded and humiliated driver of a rich man's car to becoming a rich businessman himself. The tale is told in a racy style with much bitter humour. Balram advises the Chinese premier not to dip into the revered waters of the river Ganga 'unless you want your mouth full of faeces, straw, soggy parts of human bodies, buffalo carrion and several different kinds of industrial acids.' The characters are lightly sketched but very entertaining in their awfulness.

I especially liked Balram's sentimental boss, Mr Ashok, and his posh wife, Pinky Madam.

When you reach the end of the story and come up for a breath of fresh air, you will have to decide whether you like and/or empathise with the White Tiger. Is he right that social mobility in India is only achieved by outdoing the rich at their own criminal game? Dorothy? *I don't know that it matters what we think. Balram pulls you into his car and makes you ride along with him, like him or not. It's like* Crime and Punishment, *only without the punishment. I think it's a truly original and disturbing book. And I loved Pinky Madam, too!*

The Whitbread Prize

The Whitbread Prize, now rebadged as the Costa Prize, chooses its overall book of the year from the best in five categories: novel, first novel, poetry, biography and children's book.

In 2001, the winner was a children's book which soon became very popular with adults, too. *THE AMBER SPYGLASS* is the final part of a trilogy called *His Dark Materials*. If you haven't already, we recommend that you read the whole thing!

The three parts are *Northern Lights, The Subtle Knife* and *The Amber Spyglass*. If you haven't read it yet, a wonderful experience awaits you. If you haven't heard of it before, where have you been? And let me tell you all about it at once.

Philip Pullman originally wrote this trilogy for children, but it has been enjoyed just as much by its many grown-up admirers. I was hooked from Volume One, page one, and never had any sense that I was reading a children's book. Indeed, young children might find it quite scary. So what is it all about? Well, it's a fantasy about characters who live in a number of parallel worlds, including our own. The heroine, Lyra Belaqua (aged 11) lives in Oxford, which I know quite well in my own world. But, as I read the book, it began to dawn on me that Lyra's Oxford and indeed Lyra's world has developed differently and is in some ways still medieval as well as magical. The first thing to notice is that every character has a *daemon*, a sort of alter ego in the shape of an animal, always of the opposite gender, who is their constant companion. When you are a child your daemon can metamorphose instantly to become any one of a whole range of creatures – birds, insects or mammals – according to your mood. When you grow up, it stabilises in one form to match your character. Lyra lives at Jordan College as a sort of ward, under the protection of her uncle, Lord Asriel, who is 'said to be involved in high politics, secret exploration and distant warfare.' As Lyra eavesdrops on the adults' conversation, there is talk of a strange version of science which is mixed up with theology, just as it was in Newton's time. Lyra soon realises that dirty work is afoot, that grown-ups are not to be trusted, and that the future not just of Oxford but of the whole universe is at stake. God (known as 'The Authority') is still in his heaven, but he seems to have succumbed to a celestial form of Alzheimer's disease, and an unscrupulous Regent is in charge of the Kingdom. Lyra meets all sorts of strange but astonishingly believable characters, including flying witches, polar bears who wear armour (which they make themselves) and an array of horrible beings such as Cliff-Ghasts and Spectres which make Tolkien's monsters seem quite tame. She also meets and eventually falls in adolescent first-love with Will, a boy of 13 or so. And Will acquires a special knife which can cut a window between one world and another . . .

Philip Pullman's imagination is inexhaustible, and his writing achieves an emotional intensity which can be deeply moving. If you would like another opinion, here is a review from a junior reader which I found on the Amazon website:

> I've re-read the books so many times i practically know some parts by heart. It deals with many issues, including human nature partly. Plus it is agreed by all i know that having a daemon would be the best thing ever.

The Whitbread Book of the Year 2003 was a great and unusual novel which you probably read at the time. It was of course Mark Haddon's *THE CURIOUS INCIDENT OF THE DOG IN THE NIGHT-TIME.*

I love to read a story told in the first person by someone who sounds a little bit strange and secretive. How about this for an introduction?

> My name is Christopher John Francis Boone. I know all the countries of the world and their capital cities and every prime number up to 7507.

Christopher is 15. He is very good at maths and logical puzzles and has an excellent memory. But he finds it very hard to tell what other people are thinking and feeling, and he has behavioural problems. These include not talking to people for a long time, not liking to be touched, and screaming or smashing things when he is angry and confused. Christopher seems to have Asperger's syndrome or something like it. But because we see everything from his point of view, it's the rest of the world which seems strange and unpredictable. In the first chapter, Christopher finds next door's dog lying dead with a garden fork sticking out of his body. This discovery propels him to start a Sherlock Holmes type investigation in which he tries to solve the mystery and find the identity of the murderer. This is difficult, because no one takes kindly to having an Aspergerian boy-detective going around asking awkward questions. Christopher's long-suffering father doesn't like it, and neither do the police. But Christopher persists and eventually finds himself embarking on a perilous solo train journey to London to track down his missing mother and solve some of the mysteries of his own life. In the course of telling his story, Christopher also helps us to understand how his mind works and why negotiating with 'normal' people is so difficult for him. Along the way he entertains us with diagrams, maps, puzzles and mathematical curiosities. Mark Haddon has written a really original and enjoyable book in a unique style. From the outside, Christopher appears to be cold, distant and definitely weird. But because he is allowed to tell his own story, he becomes a likeable, even lovable person.

**Now we move on to 2004, in which the Whitbread Book of the Year was
SMALL ISLAND by Andrea Levy.**

Andrea Levy was born in London to Jamaican parents, and this book tells us a lot about the experience of the West Indians who came to Britain in the 1940s. Hortense is a well brought up Jamaican girl who arrives in London in 1948 to be reunited with her husband Gilbert. Gilbert has been in the RAF, and after the war he is very anxious to return to England. Hortense lends him the money for a passage on the *Empire Windrush* in 1948. This was the boat that brought the first wave of black nurses and bus conductors to London, and the fare was apparently 28 pounds 10 shillings. To be honest, Hortense has only married Gilbert so that she will be able to come to London herself, live in a nice house with a bell that goes ding-a-ling, and get a post as a teacher. Unhappily, the reality of post-war London is disappointing. She finds Gilbert living in one room in a tall shabby house in conditions of squalor that her Jamaican family would never tolerate. Everything in the room is covered with a layer of dirt that leaves black marks on the fingers of her white gloves. However, the landlady, Queenie, is quite friendly and seems to be one of the few Londoners without a fear of 'darkies.' The fourth major character, completing the quartet, is Queenie's very conventional up-tight husband

Bernard, who has been missing since the end of the war. I hope I'm not giving too much away if I say we don't meet him until later. The story keeps flashing back to an unspecified period called 'Before' and then forward again to 1948. I found this disconcerting at first, until I realised what Andrea Levy was doing structurally. Each of the 'Before' sections is narrated by one of the four main characters, and this gives them each a chance to tell us about their background and upbringing. Wartime experiences dominate the recollections of everyone except Hortense. Gilbert spends the war in England and is shocked by the segregation of black American soldiers from their white comrades. He goes to a cinema with Queenie and there is a riot when American GIs insist that he sits in the back row reserved for the 'coloured' clients. We hear how Queenie survived the Blitz and eventually how her husband Bernard fared in India (his racist tendency only got worse). The story reaches a climax when Bernard suddenly reappears in the house and insists that the black lodgers (Gilbert and Hortense) are evicted. I shall leave you to relish the surprising end to the story yourselves. *Small Island* is an absorbing read and would be an excellent choice to take on holiday. Andrea gives each narrator a distinctive voice, and even the rather obnoxious Bernard evoked some empathy from me, given everything he had been through. And I feel I know much more about the background of the older generation of West Indian people who have been my patients for 30 years.

Now here is a book that Dorothy and I both raved about. It's the novel that won the Costa (formerly Whitbread) Prize in 2007. It's by AL Kennedy and it is simply called *DAY*.

'Day' is the surname of Alfred Day, a young man of about 25, only five foot four, an ex-RAF tail-gunner and very troubled. The year is 1949, and Alfred is working as a film extra in Germany where they are trying to recreate scenes of a prisoner-of-war camp. There's a rather unpleasant fellow there called Vasyl, who claims to be Ukrainian. He keeps trying to be friendly, but Alfred would rather hit him. Alfred has been in a real POW camp, so why would he want to repeat the experience? The fact is that his wartime memories are still churning around sickeningly in his mind – 'bad thoughts getting clever with him.' He seems to be trying to find himself, but first he has to deal with his flashbacks – the sights, sounds and smells, and the slippery feeling of his comrades' blood on the floor of the aeroplane. The book gives you a seat inside a Lancaster as it throbs and shudders across the North Sea to set Hamburg on fire. You will also get a seat inside Alfred's mind, and it will be a bumpy ride, because his thoughts and memories tumble over each other in a chaotic way. Mostly he seems to be talking to himself, but you will get used to that.

In fact the memories are not all bad. It was good learning how to be a gunner and finding your rightful place in the rear turret of the great bomber. You liked being a member of the crew, that little group of seven, each with a job to do under the protective leadership of your Skipper. You picked each other out intuitively because you felt the others were people you could bear to live with, and maybe die with. Alfred needed a new family because his childhood had not been happy. He loved his mother, but his dad used to knock her about, making Alfred want to kill him. One of those dark things inside him is the knowledge that his job is to kill people, and it gives him some pleasure. The unsavoury Vasyl in the mock POW camp seems to want to remind him of this disturbing part of himself.

On a brighter note, Alfred does manage to find love with Joyce, a married woman whom he meets during an air raid in London. Their scenes together and her letters are beautifully written.

Reading *Day* made me think of the Powell and Pressburger film *A Matter of Life and Death* (1946), in which David Niven is seen trying to fly home in a crippled Lancaster with his parachute gone and all the rest of the crew dead. I wonder if that film was the inspiration for the book. I became so fascinated with bombers that I visited the RAF Museum in Hendon to see what a real Lancaster looked like. They have one suspended in a vast hangar – an awesome sight with its guns and its Plexiglas astrodomes and its yawning empty bomb bay. But they wouldn't let me climb inside.

Sorry, Dorothy, this fascination with bombers is obviously a boy thing that you must find very tedious. *Actually no, John. I love the RAF Museum. If I'd known you were going I'd have come with you. And have you forgotten that AL Kennedy's 'A' stands for Alison and she is a woman?* Dorothy, you're right again.

THE SECRET SCRIPTURE by Sebastian Barry (2008) is the one we were betting on for the 2008 Man Booker Prize. It made the short list, but was beaten by The White Tiger. However, it went on to win the 2008 Costa Prize for Book of the Year.

This is a wonderful novel by a great Irish writer, which is also about the life of a woman, so I shall hand you straight over to Dorothy. Thank you, John. When we open this book, we find ourselves in an ancient, crumbling psychiatric hospital in the West of Ireland. The first voice we hear is that of Roseanne, who tells us that she is 'only a thing left over, a remnant woman.' She may be 100 years old (no one knows), and she has been a patient in the hospital since 1957. Nevertheless, Roseanne's mind is sharp and she is engaged in writing a 'Testimony of Herself', which we are privileged to be able to read. Meanwhile the chief psychiatrist, Dr Grene, is also writing a diary. The hospital is about to be closed, and he is concerned about the fate of the older inhabitants, particularly Roseanne, who he thinks was probably never mentally ill in the first place. Dr Grene has his own problems with his estranged and seriously unwell wife, who is avoiding diagnosis and treatment.

So what about Roseanne's life? Is it interesting? And how did she get to be incarcerated in this place? Have patience, John, I'm coming to all that. She has had an amazing and terrible life. Her beloved father was keeper of the Catholic cemetery in Sligo, despite being a Presbyterian. It was the time just after the Civil War in the 1920s. We still don't like to talk about those days, with brother killing brother and people betraying each other and all that. There is a dramatic scene when some IRA boys bring a dead comrade to the cemetery for burial. Twelve-year-old Roseanne is sent to fetch the priest. Some government soldiers also appear. Shots are fired, and the rebel men are wounded and arrested. Poor Roseanne is wrongly accused of tipping off the soldiers. When the sinister priest, Father Gaunt, who will become Roseanne's cruel tormentor and nemesis, sacks her father from his post as grave keeper, life goes rapidly downhill. But there are some better times. Roseanne meets young Tom McNulty, who is the bandleader at the Café Cairo. They fall quickly in love and get married. But then the poor girl is accused of adultery because she goes to meet one of those IRA men on the local mountain – although nothing happens, believe me. And that rotten priest, heaven forgive me for saying so, gets the marriage annulled. It's so unfair! *You are getting really involved here, Dorothy.* I am so! But that's only the beginning of her troubles. Maybe I shouldn't tell any more. I'll just say that there are some amazing scenes that will have you on the edge of your seat with shivers running up and down your back. Sebastian Barry writes in a way that is thrilling and moving. He is quite a poet, if you ask me. *I have heard that the book is also a kind of history of Ireland. Would you agree with that?* I would. It's a very sad history of all the ignorance and cruelty that was visited on poor innocent people and especially on women. But things are better now, thank goodness. And even the book has a surprise happy ending that had me hugging myself, although I was thinking, come on now Sebastian, could this really happen? You so want to believe it could. This is a lovely book, a real treasure.

The Orange Prize 2005

This prize, somewhat controversially, is for women novelists only. Dorothy, why should that be necessary in this age of equality between the sexes?

We are not yet as equal as you might think, John. Did you notice that the short list for the 2008 Man Booker Prize contained only one woman author? Although women no longer have to give themselves a male nom de plume like George Eliot or the Brontës to begin with, the literary establishment still seems to privilege men. So we need the Orange Prize, and long may it continue!

OK, well let's talk about the winner of the 2005 Orange Prize, **WE NEED TO TALK ABOUT KEVIN** by Lionel Shriver. Having heard what it was about I embarked on it with some anxiety, but my duty to deliver a report from the front line to the Green Bookshop's customers kept me going. After a rather slow start (putting it down to read other books, the way you do), I was eventually gripped and full of admiration. So what is the problem with Kevin and why do we need to talk about him? I hate to have to tell you this, but Kevin is the perpetrator of an American high-school massacre. And from the day of his birth his mother, Eva, found him not only hard to understand but impossible to love. The story is told in the form of a series of letters written by Eva to her husband, from whom she is separated. The nature of this separation only becomes clear in the final electrifying chapters. In the letters, Eva describes her difficult life in a community where everyone knows she is the mother of a teenage monster who is responsible for the deaths of seven of their children. She recalls her reluctance to have a child in the first place, and then the birth of Kevin, who rejects her breast along with just about everything else she has to offer. He screams constantly whenever his mother is present, but shuts up for his father, who desperately tries to see his son as a normal child. And Eva tries her best to love him, too. But the atrocious Kevin progresses remorselessly from a horrendous baby to a sarcastic four-year-old who mocks his parents, destroys his toys and seems to have no capacity or need for affection. He is cruel and heartless, and his mother is certain that he was responsible for his timid little sister's unfortunate loss of an eye. We meet the 17-year-old Kevin during Eva's regular and dutiful visits to him in the juvenile prison. He seems to be enjoying the experience, and when his mother cautiously asks if the other inmates treat him well, his reply is 'They fucking worship me!' That's Kevin for you. His utterances are crisp and articulate, and I even began to have a sneaking affection for him. That is until the shock horror revelation of what actually happened in the school on that fateful Thursday – which, obviously, I am not going to reveal. We are offered no explanation for Kevin. He is not autistic or brain damaged, and his parents did their best to love and care for him. He is just plain vicious, with a black sense of humour. Like his parents, you may find Kevin hard to live with. But Lionel Shriver writes well with plenty of wit and shrewd observation. And did I mention suspense? So please give the book a try. It will bring enjoyment tempered with unease.

CHAPTER 3

Great books that should
have won prizes

Here we have a collection of really outstanding novels published between 2002 and 2008. They are all a joy to read and even to read over again. None of them won prizes, but they are all awarded the Green Bookshop Gold Star Prize. And they are all in stock!

CLOUD ATLAS by David Mitchell (2004)

David Mitchell's *Cloud Atlas* was one of the most exciting books to arrive in the Green Bookshop in 2004. But first a word of warning for those of you who are wary of books that play tricks with time, speak in different voices and have six different plots. This book does all of those things and more, but once you get the hang of it, I think you will really enjoy it. Yes, there are six different stories, but they don't follow each other in the normal way. The first one gets to an exciting point about halfway through and then breaks off. The next story does the same, and so on, until you get to the sixth one, which is complete. The other stories then finish themselves off, starting with number five, so that the last thing you read is the conclusion of the first one. Think of it as like one of those Russian dolls, each inside the next one, with a solid doll in the middle.

Now I'll tell you a bit about the stories. The first one is set in the early nineteenth century, and is told by an American lawyer who suffers from a mysterious illness while on a sea voyage in the South Pacific. Then we jump to Belgium in the 1930s, and read the letters of an unscrupulous young musician who is sponging off a retired English composer. Tale number three is an

American thriller such as you might pick up at an airport bookshop (although you'd be lucky to find one as good as this). Then we are back in present-day England, reading the memoirs of an elderly publisher, an engaging old rogue who finds himself committed by his brother to an old people's home from which he engineers an ingenious escape (echoes of *One Flew Over the Cuckoo's Nest* and also *Jeffrey Bernard is Unwell*). Story number five is set in a dystopic future, and is told in the form of an interview for the Archives, by its heroine, a genetically engineered 'fabricant' who is programmed to spend her short life as a server in a fast-food restaurant, but manages to escape and begin to understand what sort of society has produced her. All sorts of new words enter the language here, and we have to think hard about concepts like free will and happiness and mind control. Imagine *Brave New World* meets *1984* with a strong dash of Ridley Scott's *Blade Runner*. The core story is breathtakingly original in both language and concept. It's a post-global-disaster scenario in which a small peaceful farming community is being menaced by very scary mounted bandits called the Kona. They are saved from extinction by a visitor from another group of survivors, called the Prescients, who have retained some knowledge of history and pre-holocaust technology. This chapter reaches an exciting and moving conclusion that left me well satisfied and ready to close the book. Then I realised that I still had the outer five stories to finish! Questions inevitably arise. What themes link these apparently disparate stories? What is the point of the Russian doll structure? What makes it such a brilliant and original book?

A few tentative answers before you read it and draw your own conclusions. There are several tenuous plot links between the stories, including a mysterious comet-shaped birthmark that the principal characters seem to pass on to each other. Then I notice that the stories are all about desperate escapes from situations in which gentle, emotionally intelligent beings are being exploited, enslaved or even exterminated by ruthless aggressors. However, the initial threat may be quite subtle, and it can be difficult to know who are your friends and who are your enemies. The wise Prescient woman sums up the moral issues for humanity in a few well-chosen words on page 318. Whatever you think about the book's message, I have to add that the writing is brilliant throughout, and incredibly versatile. The style in each story is a kind of parody of typical examples of its genre, and in the two inner stories the language evolves and mutates with amazing flexibility. I'm reminded of James Joyce's *Ulysses*, but don't let that put you off. This book is not difficult to read, and it's truly remarkable.

BRICK LANE by Monica Ali (2003)

In the Green Bookshop's opinion, *Brick Lane* by Monica Ali was the best novel of its year and should definitely be on your reading list. You may have been to Brick Lane in London's East End for a curry, but have you ever wondered what it would be like to be whisked from a village in Bangladesh to a flat in Tower Hamlets? This is the fate of Monica Ali's heroine, Nazneen, who has been brought to London as a bride at the age of 17. Nazneen began life as a near stillborn baby who was 'left to her fate' instead of being rushed to hospital. On her fifth day of life, she decided to clamp on to her mother's nipple and survive. In East End London, fate decrees that she will be the wife of a man called Chanu, who is 40 years old and has a face like a frog. Nazneen is a quiet girl, but she takes a keen interest in her surroundings and tries to understand what life in the Bangladeshi community is all about. Fortunately, her husband, although obese and unappetising, is very kind and gentle. He is a graduate of Dhaka University and also has an Open University degree, but somehow professional success eludes him and he ends up as a minicab driver. Sadly, their first child dies in infancy, but they go on to have two spirited daughters who naturally take a keen interest in English youth culture. Their father, on the other hand, yearns to take his family back to Bangladesh if only he can save up the money.

At first, Nazneen tries to accept her life the way it is. She cooks for her husband, she pares his corns and cuts his toenails, she looks after her girls, and she talks to the other women in the block. Chanu buys her a sewing machine and she starts to earn some money doing piecework. Then she falls for Karim, the young man who brings her bundles of jeans to sew, and they start having an affair. If you are wondering how the situation will be resolved, I will say only that Nazneen suddenly realises that she can make some important decisions about her own future. Although Monica Ali has been hailed as a brilliant whizz-kid of a writer, there is nothing flashy about her style. She tells her story in simple straightforward prose which is easy to read. But every so often she comes up with a beautiful image which gleams like a jewel, or a little insight that makes you nod your head in agreement.

STAR OF THE SEA by Joseph O'Connor (2003)

The year is 1847 and we are in the middle of the terrible Irish famine. The 'Star of the Sea' is a leaky old paddle steamer heading across the Atlantic on a 26-day voyage from Ireland to New York. Her steerage deck is crammed with over 400 starving immigrants who are desperately hoping to start a new life as Americans – if they can survive the journey. Travelling in much greater comfort, there are also 15 first-class passengers, including the young Lord Kingscourt and his family, and an American journalist of liberal sympathies called Dixon. The journalist is having an affair with Lady Kingscourt, while her husband has designs on their maidservant Mary, whom he has known since they were children. Every night a strange ragged man with a scarred face and a deformed foot walks up and down the ship from stem to stern and back again. His mission is to murder Lord Kingscourt before the ship reaches New York. The story is told by Dixon, the journalist, with interpolated extracts from the Captain's log. This records, among other details, the grim tally of passengers dying from hunger and disease every single day. As the ship ploughs its way across the ocean, we learn more and more about the personal histories of all the main characters whose lives overlap and intersect each other. Mary the maid's family were tenants on Lord Kingscourt's Galway estate, and the young master was her first love. Pius Mulvey, the mysterious contract killer, also began life on the same estate. He has subsequently had a colourful career as a petty criminal in London, culminating in a brutally exciting escape from Newgate Prison. And now he is planning to murder his former landlord. O'Connor's writing is vivid and convincing, and he enlists our sympathy for all the characters, including the psychopathic Mulvey. He also sets the fictional story firmly in its historical context. *Star of the Sea* is an enjoyable and engrossing read, which also made me appreciate the catastrophic scale of the Irish famine, in which a million people died as a result of greed, incompetence and indifference.

THAT THEY MAY FACE THE RISING SUN by John McGahern (2002)

After that rather disturbing book, you might need a more calming Irish experience to follow. If the title is a puzzle, I promise that you will know exactly what it means by the time you have finished the book. I'll read you the first paragraph just to give you an idea of McGahern's tranquil, limpid style:

> The morning was clear. There was no wind on the lake. When the bells rang out for Mass, the strokes trembled on the water, they had the entire world to themselves.

So we are in remote, rural Ireland and we are going to spend time with the people who live by the lake. Our hosts are a retired couple in late middle age called the Ruttledges. They spend their time pottering about, gossiping with the neighbours, doing a bit of farming and watching the seasons go round. At first it seems as if nothing is going to happen, and then you find yourself getting really interested in the characters who drop in and involve the Ruttledges in their affairs. Gradually they reveal themselves and their interrelationships to the visiting reader. They are all slightly strange, and some of them have had desperately lonely lives, but they have resilience and plenty of humour. I say nothing happens, but we get to watch calves and lambs being born, we manage to get the meadows mown for hay before the weather breaks, and we go to a wedding and a cattle auction. We have a daring discussion with the local IRA man, whose house is always watched by two detectives (sometimes three). Towards the end of the book, the narrative focuses on the last days of another exile, who has come home to Ireland after spending most of his adult life working in England. After showing his old friends that he is still an ace darts player, he dies suddenly, and the community gathers to lay him out, bury him and mourn him.

That's about it, really. It seems very simple, so what makes it so special? I think it must be the quality of the writing, which never calls attention to itself, but is so quietly and magically effective that you feel you have been completely drawn into the community, and when you get to the end you will feel sorry that you have to leave.

OLD SCHOOL by Tobias Wolff (2004)

Now for those of you who feel it is time to move on from Harry Potter and Hogwarts, let me recommend a novel called *Old School* by Tobias Wolff. It is set in a posh boys-only boarding school situated somewhere in the Eastern United States. In the sixth form, the boys' overriding interest is in writing. Three times a year, the headmaster invites a famous writer to visit the school and judge a literary competition. The boy who enters the best poem or story in a competition wins a private interview with the celebrity guest. The famous writers are real ones, and the words Tobias Wolff imagines for them are so convincing that you really believe you have met them, too. First comes the poet Robert Frost, who is very genial about a poem that he wrongly believes is trying to send up his own style. Next, causing a considerable stir, is the ultra-right-wing American novelist Ayn Rand, who has a Nietzschean belief in the right of the strong 'creative' man or woman to disregard the welfare of the 'common herd.' She chooses a sci-fi story in which a flying saucer crewed by super-cows tries to rescue their fellow cows on earth from a life of slavery and slaughter. She thinks that it's a satire on the stupidity of the herd, although its boy author intended it as a plea for vegetarianism. Our unnamed hero gets very excited when he hears that Ernest Hemingway is to be the next guest. He worships Hemingway, and tries to get inspiration by copying out the great man's own short stories. Then he comes across a story in the magazine of a neighbouring girls' school, which is so good that he is devastated. It begins with the schoolgirl narrator picking up a lipstick-stained cigarette end because she is desperate for a smoke, and hoping that no one has seen her. She reveals herself to be an unhappy person who has to tell lies to ingratiate herself with her snobbish friends. Our narrator immediately recognises himself in this character. Here is a writer who, just like his idol Hemingway, is not afraid to let herself be seen as she really is. He copies the story, changes only a few details, and enters it for the competition under his own name. Of course his deception is discovered, and there are consequences which I shall not reveal here. One of the main themes of the book is the way people are afraid to tell the truth about themselves because of their fear of being rejected socially or professionally, and their need to be loved and accepted. It's quite short, and it's so beautifully and carefully written that as soon as I had finished it I had to read it all over again.

MIDDLESEX by Jeffrey Eugenides (2002)

This is a nice thick heart-warming family saga, which spreads generously over three generations and takes in some of the major upheavals of the twentieth century. If you also like genetics, Greek food and gender identity problems, this is definitely the book for you. It's called *Middlesex*, and I should really have promoted it when it won the Pulitzer Prize in 2003. Somehow it was overlooked at the time, but I am all the more eager to do it justice now. The book has a wonderful opening paragraph. Actually it consists of three paragraphs and a single line, which act like an overture, rehearsing the main themes. It begins:

> I was born twice: first as a baby girl, on a remarkably smogless Detroit day in January of 1960, and then again, as a teenage boy, in an emergency room near Petoskey, Michigan, in August of 1974. Specialised readers may have come across me in Dr Peter Luce's study, 'Gender identity in 5-Alpha-Reductase Pseudohermaphrodites' published in the Journal of Pediatric Endocrinology in 1975.

Cal or Callie (as our hero is variously called, according to whether she is boy or girl) then narrates the whole of the saga, although it starts several decades before she is born. She begins with her grandparents, who are living in a Greek village in Asia Minor (look it up). A young man known as Lefty (short for Eleutherios) complains to his sister Desdemona that there are no eligible girls in the village for him to marry. When the Turkish army suddenly invades, they have to flee for their lives, and end up in America. During the transatlantic voyage, brother and sister fall in love with each other and are married by the ship's captain. They know this is not really allowed – but what the hell, nobody knows who they are. Are you ready for some genetics? The happy young couple are blissfully unaware that they are each carrying a recessive gene on the fifth chromosome that blocks the production of an enzyme called 5-alpha reductase. Without this enzyme, a boy baby can't produce dihydrotestosterone, his testes won't descend, and he is brought up as a girl. No one suspects anything until puberty, when regular testosterone starts to squirt from those hidden gonads producing disturbing gender ambiguity. But this all comes later. To begin with we can enjoy a thrilling and colourful narrative as the emigrants are welcomed to Detroit by their cousin and her husband. Lefty soon becomes a real American, although Desdemona remains firmly attached to her Greek heritage. Lefty works briefly on the Ford assembly line and then, with the help of his cousin-in-law, gets a more exciting job as a bootlegger. Desdemona teaches silkworm cultivation to an organisation called The Nation of Islam.

They have a son called Milton, who woos his cousin Tessie with a seductive clarinet (touching her intimately with the bell of the instrument as he plays). All this incurable incest enables those recessive family genes to cosy up together, too, and that is how our heroine Callie gets to be born a hermaphrodite. There's a nice account of her girlhood (tall, awkward and sensitive), culminating in an overwhelming crush on a gorgeous, red haired, pale-skinned, freckled female classmate. Their innocent lovemaking is enhanced by Callie's unusual genital development. Then the family doctor discovers Callie's secret. Her distraught parents rush her off to the Gender Identity Clinic. Now there's some more science, with a fascinating discussion of the various factors that determine gender. Dr Luce thinks that Callie should remain a girl, and proposes surgery, but Cal has other ideas. I'll stop there because maybe I've said too much already. The plot is always intriguing, but the writing is good, too, and there's plenty of humour. So please take a copy of *Middlesex*. You will have a great read, and learn a lot about intersexuality, including, most importantly, how it feels to belong to a third gender that no one finds acceptable.

SUITE FRANÇAISE by Irène Némirovsky (2006)

Now let's look at an intriguing French novel. No, don't run away, it has been translated. Have you ever wondered what it would be like to have your country invaded? What was it like to be in Paris in the summer of 1940 when the Germans arrived? *Suite Française* is a remarkable account of that time by someone who lived through it, but sadly did not survive the war and the Holocaust. Irène Némirovsky was born into a Jewish family in Kiev in 1903. In 1918 the family fled from the Russian Revolution to France, where Irène lived happily until the outbreak of war. After the fall of France in 1940, she began work on what was to have been a grand five-part saga about the war. Only the first two parts were finished when she and her husband were arrested by the Nazis and taken to Auschwitz, where they died. However, their two daughters were hidden from the police by their teacher, and managed to escape. The elder daughter, Denise, took with her the leather-bound notebook in which she had observed her mother writing. For years Denise and her sister couldn't bear to look at the notebook, but finally the tiny writing was deciphered with the aid of a magnifying glass, and *Suite Française* was eventually published in France in 2004. An English translation was published in 2006.

What we have in the English edition is the completed first two parts, Irène's notes for the whole five-part scheme, and some of her letters and the story I have just briefly told you. Part One is called 'Storm in June.' The first chapter is an evocation of that hot June evening when the Parisians heard the news on their radios that the Germans were shortly to march into their city. Then we are introduced to a number of middle-class families and individuals as they make their preparations to flee down south with as many of their worldly goods as they can cram into their cars. First there's the supercilious Pericand family, consisting of mother, father, two grown up sons, three younger children, wheelchair-bound grandfather, nanny, servants and Albert the cat. Then we meet the writer Gabriel Corte, who is anxious to save his manuscripts, the 60-year-old art collector who carefully packs up his collection of priceless porcelain, and the middle-aged couple who work for a bank and are worried about what has happened to their soldier son in the defeated French army.

Apart from the last two, just about everyone we meet behaves badly. In their panic-stricken flight they think only of themselves, quarrelling over the limited supplies of food and accommodation. The art collector even steals a can of petrol from the car of a young married couple. Along the roads and in the towns through which they pass they are periodically bombed and strafed by German aircraft. Some of the more obnoxious characters meet a suitably unpleasant fate. There are not many examples of people behaving with decency, but there are a few. Seventeen-year-old Hubert Pericand sets off bravely on his bicycle to enlist, and after joining a group of soldiers and coming under fire, he manages to find his way back to his family. 'Everywhere you look,' he says to himself, 'chaos, cowardice, vanity and ignorance.' Would we have behaved any better if Hitler had crossed the channel, I wonder.

In Part Two ('Dolce'), the German Occupation is fully established. We are in a village whose inhabitants are finding out what it's like to have the soldiers who have conquered their country living in their house. What are they like? Surprisingly, they are ordinary, healthy young men, and for the most part they are well behaved. One of the officers is attracted to Lucille, whose husband is away in the army, or is perhaps a prisoner. A civilised friendship develops in which they talk about culture as they walk in the garden. There is a mutual physical attraction, but when the young officer makes a move, Lucille repels him (thankfully!). There are some humorous moments when the local aristocrats present the Germans with a list of articles they would like returned from their occupied manor house, including a valuable tea service and Papa's spare set of false teeth! There is some excitement when one of the farmers shoots a German and has to go into hiding. Finally, one day, the Germans suddenly disappear, having been called away to fight on the Russian front.

Suite Française is brilliantly written, with sure and precise drawing of character, sharp satire and evocative descriptions. Most of the people behave disgracefully, but you can't help feeling a sneaking sympathy for them, because their creator understands them so well. The cat Albert has a nice chapter all to himself. This is a great book, probably a classic. Make sure it goes in your suitcase.

THE LAY OF THE LAND by Richard Ford (2006)

Now I'd like to share with you a new discovery of mine – the American writer Richard Ford. I have just been enjoying his latest novel, *The Lay of the Land*, which I'll tell you about in a minute. Some of you may know about Richard Ford already, in which case you will have to bear with me while I go over his history. His first really successful book was *The Sportswriter* (1986). The central character, Frank Bascombe, then reappeared in a second book called *Independence Day* (1995), which won the Pulitzer Prize. I'm ashamed to say I didn't read either of them, and all the ballyhoo just passed me by. Finally, in 2006 the Frank Bascombe trilogy was completed with *The Lay of the Land*, which is the one I have read and am now going to tell you about.

Frank Bascombe is now aged 55 and has reached what he calls the Permanent Period of life. This is the time when you can feel reassured that you have a few achievements to your credit and that nothing much more is going to happen in your life, but it will go on quite pleasantly being the same (until the end). Or as Frank puts it, 'You realise you can't completely fuck everything up anymore, since so much of your life is on the books already.' Younger readers may find this feeling difficult to understand, but at 65, believe me, it rings a few bells. So what is Frank's situation? He is a real estate agent selling houses in a pleasant seafront town in New Jersey. He has prostate cancer which is being treated with implanted radio-iodine seeds. He and his first wife lost a son and were divorced shortly afterwards. His second wife of eight years, Sally, has just left him to go and live in Mull, Scotland with her first husband, Wally, who was presumed dead but has annoyingly turned up alive. He has two surviving children – the sympathetic, possibly lesbian Clarissa and the strange, aggressive, needy, possibly autistic Paul. During the course of the book not much happens. Well no, that's not true, all sorts of things happen, like nearly selling a house, getting into a clumsy brawl in a bar, going to an old friend's funeral, spending a night in the car and trying to understand his children and wives. And that's just a selection of the events in this sprawling 725-page book. There's also a big shock to shatter your complacency near the end (which I shall not reveal).

So why did Richard Ford make such a big impression on me? It is because his writing is so brilliant. Frank tells his story in the form of a rambling conversation with himself. He follows every train of thought wherever it's going, he observes the changing landscape and architecture of his New Jersey home, he broods on relationships, on life, old age and death. The style owes something to James Joyce and Marcel Proust, but the laconic voice is more like that of Garrison Keillor. I should add that Frank's story of himself is very sharp and funny, thanks to Mr Ford's wry sense of humour and his wonderful way with words. Yes, it's a long read, but once you make friends with Frank you will want him to go on being your companion for page after page. Please give it a try. Meanwhile I shall be ordering copies of the first two books. Then I need to go off somewhere for a fortnight where no one can find me, to read them.

IF NOBODY SPEAKS OF REMARKABLE THINGS by Jon McGregor (2003)

This is a very original and exciting first novel by the up-and-coming Jon McGregor, who lives in Nottingham. The book tells the story of a street and an accident that happens there, and it's also the self-told story of a young woman who lives in the street and was loved by a boy with itchy eyes, although she never really knew him. The intriguing first chapter urges us to listen to the singing of the city. We hear all the different noises and hold our breath in the short night-time silence when everything is still. Then we zoom in on a young couple dancing in the car park of an Indian restaurant. It's a magical beginning. In the chapters that follow, the young woman's personal story alternates with the voice of an all-seeing narrator who observes what goes on up and down the street and tells us about the people who live in each and every house. At Number 19, there's an Indian couple with twin boys who love playing cricket and are rather mischievous. They have a younger sister who would like to join in the cricket, but they won't let her. At Number 20, there's an old couple who were married during the Second World War and are still in love. We are privileged to listen to some of their recollections, like the day the man came back from the army looking for her and she said 'I'm right behind you.' Sadly, he is now coughing up bloodstained sputum and the young doctor has told him, in her euphemistic way, that things are not 100 per cent as she would like them, but he hasn't worked out how to tell his wife yet. There are students at Number 17. There's a whole street full of interesting people, and I found it helpful to draw myself a sketch map and label it so that I knew where everybody was living. At Number 18 lives the boy with dry sore eyes who collects things and who had a blissful afternoon with the girl with short hair and square glasses from Number 22, but she was too drunk to remember him. She is the young woman who tells her own story in alternate chapters. It's about her parents and how she came to be pregnant, and her relationship with Michael, who is the twin brother of the boy with dry eyes who loved her with a hopeless longing. There's a fantastic chapter describing a rainstorm that sweeps down the street. And then the accident, described in slow motion, which is the reason why everyone in the street remembers that day. Jon McGregor writes like a poet. His descriptions are breathtaking, and he has also created a whole collection of memorable characters, some of whom we get to know in some depth. By the time I reached the end (which is quite hopeful) I felt as if I lived there myself.

THE ENCHANTRESS OF FLORENCE by Salman Rushdie (2008)

This novel made the long list for the 2008 Booker Prize and then disappeared. But it definitely gets a Green Bookshop prize.

Salman Rushdie, that old silver-tongued wordsmith, has written a brilliant historical fantasy which sweeps us from Mughal India to Renaissance

Florence and back again. The first chapter paints a gorgeous picture of a glowing lake, appearing golden in the sunset. We are outside the palace-city of Sikri, the capital of the sixteenth-century Mughal Emperor Akbar, a man of fearsome power and considerable wisdom. Travelling to Sikri to meet him is a young Italian with long yellow hair, wearing a long coat 'made up of bright-coloured harlequins of leather.' The young man has a story to tell 'which could make his fortune or else cost him his life.' Sensing that he has his audience entranced, the author turns up his magic and gives us a stunning picture of the vibrant city:

> And here again with bright silk banners from red palace windows was Sikri, shimmering in the heat like an opium vision. Here at last with its strutting peacocks and dancing girls was home.

And so on. But before I get completely drunk on the writing, I had better give you an outline of the plot. The young Italian (whose real name is Niccolo Vespucci) has a tale to tell of a fabulously beautiful Mughal princess, sister of Akbar's grandfather, who was serially captured by foreign rulers and then disappeared from history. The Princess's name was Qara Köz, but we can call her Black Eyes. Niccolo also cheekily claims to be the Emperor's uncle. This improbable tale will take a long time to unfold, and the episodes are punctuated by plots, battles, elephants, seductions and other excitements.

In Part Two the scene shifts to Florence, where we meet three sex-mad adolescent boys who are trying to find mandrake roots in the woods. (Mandrake roots? Ask me later.) Two of them like travelling, while the third prefers to stay at home. One boy travels to Asia to become a mercenary soldier, and ends up in charge of the Turkish Sultan's army. The second boy grows up to become Niccolo Machiavelli, the brilliant but ultimately disappointed political adviser to the rulers of Florence. The third boy, who likes to stay at home, will end up travelling west across the ocean like his more famous cousin Amerigo. The mercenary general rescues Lady Black Eyes and carries her to Florence, where her beauty drives everyone crazy, so that she becomes the Enchantress of Florence and is known as Angelica. I don't think I mentioned that she always has with her an almost equally desirable slave girl who looks just like her and is called The Mirror. There's a lot more to tell, but I think that will do until you can get the book home. However, I must say something about the many sexy women. We are told that men are stunned by their beauty and overwhelmed with desire.

Much of this is based on the courtly love romances of Renaissance Florence, notably Ariosto's epic *Orlando Furioso*. But I am guessing that Rushdie's language is rather less refined. Some of the girls are princesses, but there also multitudes of whores who seem to be necessary to quench the Emperor's thirst. He even has an imaginary Queen, of whom all his other wives and concubines are jealous. Fancy inventing a woman and persuading everyone that she is real! How absurd is that! Of course as a man I can enjoy all this soft Eastern pornography, but I'm also a bit troubled. In a way all of the women are imaginary. They don't seem to have much of a life outside sex with the boss, and although they can exert power, it's all done through manipulation of the men. Dorothy, what do you think? You have been very quiet. Did you like the book? *I did, yes, and I know what you mean about the women. But look, isn't it written by a man? So what can you expect? We all have to be the Enchantress, or the Witch, or an adoring slave, or the People's Princess or whatever his lordship wishes. At one point, the Emperor talks of 'a man's need for a woman to tell you that you are hers and to turn your mind away from death.' It's my belief you are all of you searching for the beautiful young mothers of your childhood. Dr Freud had a point there, I think. But despite all of that, Rushdie is a dazzling writer and* The Enchantress *is a great read.* Thank you, Dorothy. It's good to have the opinion of a real woman.

And to quote Rushdie once more, 'language upon a silver tongue affords enchantment enough.'

CHAPTER 4

Two books by one writer

Ian McEwan
Atonement (2001)
Saturday (2005)

Philip Roth
The Plot Against America (2004)
Everyman (2006)

Kazuo Ishiguro
Never Let Me Go (2005)
When We Were Orphans (2000)

José Saramago
Blindness (1995)
The Year of the Death of Ricardo Reis (1984)

Sebastian Faulks
Human Traces (2005)
Engleby (2007)

In the course of reviewing many new novels, we have acquired some favourite authors and written about not one but two of their books. So it seemed a good idea to present them together and say a little about each author's literary trajectory so far. Some may have written their best books before the two you will find here. For some their greatest work is still to come. Either way you may want to keep an eye on them. And the titles here are certainly worth reading. Three of these writers are British (Ian McEwan, Sebastian Faulks and Kazuo Ishiguro), Philip Roth is American, and José Saramago is Portuguese.

IAN McEWAN was born in 1948 in Aldershot, Hampshire, but spent much of his childhood abroad in Europe and Africa. He was the first student to enrol for the MA in Creative Writing at the University of East Anglia, where his tutor was Malcolm Bradbury. His early writing is notable for its skill but also for its rather macabre subject matter. He seems to be preoccupied with murder, child abuse and perversity.

This is evident in his first short story collection, *First Love, Last Rites* (1975), and also in *The Cement Garden* (1978). The latter is about two children, brother and sister, who tell no one about the death of their mother, and keep her body in the cellar. Creepy but very compelling! Other novels followed in a similar vein. *Black Dogs* (1992) explored real-life horrors of the twentieth century. *Enduring Love* (1997) was made into a film and had a memorable balloon accident in the first chapter. Then came *Amsterdam* (1998), about a Hitchcockian murder pact which many of us found disappointing, but it won the Booker Prize that year. With *Atonement* (2001) the author seemed to mature and to observe life more broadly and with more compassion. It may be his best book to date. *Saturday* (2005) is also a great read, and so is *Chesil Beach* (2007). McEwan has also written film scripts and more recently an opera libretto for the composer Michael Berkeley.

ATONEMENT (2001)

If you have read any of McEwan's earlier books, you will know that he tends to have a dark inner world, and that he writes very well but is sometimes a bit patchy. For instance, I thought that nothing else in *Enduring Love* really lived up to the account of the balloon disaster with which the book opens. But *Atonement* is different. The writing is terrific and the characters are seen with more compassion (and a good deal of empathy). The narrative grips you tightly all the way through, and much of the excitement comes near the end before the final intriguing resolution. If this account sounds a bit thin on plot, it's because there is so much I don't want to give away.

All right then, but what is it about? We start with a well-to-do family living in a large country house in Surrey in 1935. The younger daughter, Briony, aged 13, has just written a play and is hoping to have it performed for the family with the help of her visiting cousins. We hear a lot about how it feels to be sure that you are a writer. Is Briony a sort of McEwan alter ego? I think so. Briony soon finds herself eavesdropping on a strange scene involving her elder sister, Celia, who strips down to her underwear and plunges into a fountain after a struggle with a young man called Robbie. Cecilia and Robbie fall in love. Briony passes Cecilia a rather shocking note from Robbie, after opening it and reading it first. Her jealousy (if that is what it is) leads her to commit the 'crime' for which she spends a large part of her life seeking the 'atonement' of the title.

In Part Two the scene shifts to the hinterland of Dunkirk in 1940, where we find Robbie among the British soldiers trying desperately to reach the coast, surrounded by fleeing refugees and under constant attack from the bombing and strafing of German Stuka pilots. This part of the story is vivid and often terrifying. In Part Three, Briony has enrolled as a student nurse at St Thomas's Hospital and has to deal with the incoming casualties from the Dunkirk evacuation. This part contains more horrible wounds as well as iron Nightingale discipline, and Briony has to grow up rather quickly. I'm not going to tell you any more about the plot except that the ending is really good and leaves you wondering about the relationship between truth and imagination, as well as atonement.

But before we leave *Atonement*, I simply must draw your attention to a passage on pages 92–3. Robbie has left Cambridge with a First in English Literature and is now thinking of studying medicine. In this passage he imagines himself as a doctor at 50, his study full of objects reflecting his travels and interests and the shelves crammed with all his favourite novels and poetry:

> For this was the point, surely: he would be a better doctor for having read literature. What deep readings his modified sensibility might make of human suffering, of the self-destructive folly or sheer bad luck that drives men towards ill health! Birth, death and frailty in between. Rise and fall – this was the doctor's business and it was literature's, too.

Sadly, Robbie never gets to become a doctor. I have written to Ian McEwan asking him if he ever thought about doing medicine himself.

SATURDAY (2005)

He didn't reply, but here in his next novel is the confirmation of my suspicion, which arose from reading *Atonement*, that he has a secret desire to be a doctor. His hero in *Saturday* is a consultant neurosurgeon, who is lumbered with the rather pompous name of Henry Perowne. (Why not Harry Brown? No matter.) There is more than a touch of idealisation as well as respect in McEwan's portrayal of this top-of-the-range doctor. Henry is a brilliant operator, 'renowned for his speed, his success rate and his list – he takes over three hundred cases a year.' We get a close-up view of some of these operations, with precise and accurately detailed descriptions. The author observed operations in the theatres at Queen Square over a period of two years, and he knows all the neuroanatomy that you and I have forgotten.

But Mr Perowne is not just a professional success – he also has a near perfect private life as well. His lovely wife (whom he first met when she was having a transphenoidal hypophysectomy) offers him all the love and companionship that a man could need, and he has never strayed from her warm cosy bed. His children are bright, loving and talented, too. Eighteen-year-old Theo is a brilliant blues guitarist, and Daisy, who must be about 21, has just had her first volume of poetry published. So is there something missing from our doctor's life? Or is something about to go horribly wrong? Without giving too much away, I can answer both questions with a sort of modified yes.

We follow Henry around London during the course of a single day ('Saturday'), which happens to be the day of the London protest march against the invasion of Iraq. During this Saturday we are carried around in his mind with privileged access to his thoughts and feelings. This structure reminds me strongly of James Joyce's *Ulysses*, where we follow Leopold Bloom round Dublin. Of course there are differences – Bloomsday was a Thursday, Leopold didn't do any brain surgery, and his bed companion was notoriously unfaithful. But, like Leopold, Henry does have a confrontation with a menacing opponent. During the course of his day his beautiful silver Mercedes is scraped by a red BMW driven by a man called Baxter. When the two men get out of their cars to exchange details, Henry receives a punch in the chest. He is saved from further damage because his eagle eye detects evidence in Baxter's eye movements of the early signs of Huntington's disease. You really have to be on your neurological toes to keep up with this plot. I shall say no more except to mention that the story reaches a thrilling and gripping climax when, towards the end, the two men meet again and Henry's whole family is threatened. (Don't worry, it all ends happily.) So, to return to my earlier question, what is missing from Henry Perowne's brain? First of all, he has no feeling for literature, despite plenty of coaching from his daughter. He does like to have classical music playing while he operates, but that's just treating Bach like aural wallpaper. Secondly, it occurred to me that the evil, neurologically challenged Baxter might represent the surgical superhero's missing dark side – fear of failure, insecurity, dread of humiliation and the use of violence. You don't agree? Well, it was just a speculation. Anyway, *Saturday* is exceedingly well written and a pleasure to read, with lots of extra fun for doctors.

PHILIP ROTH was born in Newark, New Jersey, USA in 1933. In a long and successful career as a novelist, he has watched through the eyes of his secular Jewish American characters the troubled course of American history in the twentieth century. Other favourite themes include the joys and sorrows of the implacable male sex drive, family life, and the struggle against death. He is also in love with literature, and his books are full of references to literary classics. He has a number of alter egos, of whom the best known is Nathan Zuckerman, also a writer and probably not very different from Philip himself.

Philip Roth can be very funny. The first book that really made him famous (and notorious) was *Portnoy's Complaint* (1959), which is all about adolescent masturbation and Jewish mothers. He is very fond of Kafka, and has written a hilarious Kafka tribute in which a professor of literature finds himself transformed into an enormous female breast. His style also makes use of a technique called amplification. This is the use of repetition with variation in order to build up the cumulative effect of his character's arguments. It can be very powerful and effective, but can be a little exhausting if overdone. Among the middle-period books I would recommend are *My Life as a Man* (1974), *The Ghost Writer* (1979) and *The Anatomy Lesson* (1983), all featuring the life and loves of Nathan Zuckerman. Then you can go on to the late trilogy *American Pastoral* (1997), *I Married a Communist* (1998) and *The Human Stain* (2000). But if you are new to Roth, you couldn't do better than to start with the following book.

THE PLOT AGAINST AMERICA (2004)

In the 1990s, Philip Roth seems to have entered a golden late middle age of inspired writing. The title of this book, *The Plot Against America*, immediately suggests 9/11 and the current climate of anxiety about terrorist attacks. However, the cover design features a one-cent US stamp heavily overprinted with a swastika, indicating that this book deals with the 1940s when Philip Roth was growing up in Newark, New Jersey.

> Fear presides over these memories, a perpetual fear. Of course no childhood is without its terrors, yet I wonder if would have been a less frightened boy if Lindbergh hadn't been president or if I hadn't been the offspring of Jews.

That's the first sentence, which sets the agenda for everything that follows. But wait a minute, who was that president again? What happened to Franklin D Roosevelt? Then we realise that Roth is offering an alternative and very disturbing history that might just have happened. Charles Lindbergh was a pilot who became a national treasure in 1927 when he made the first solo transatlantic flight from New York to Paris. Unfortunately, he then went on to become an anti-Semitic Nazi sympathiser who campaigned against American entry into the Second World War.

In Roth's nightmare scenario, Lindbergh runs for president, defeats the mighty Roosevelt and keeps America out of the war. He continues to cultivate the Nazis and invites their foreign minister, von Ribbentrop, to dine at the White House. Meanwhile, in New Jersey, life goes on. Seven year-old Philip Roth explores the complexities of family and community relationships just as he would have done with Roosevelt as president. But some things are different – and very frightening. There is a tense apprehension among the Jewish families that make up Philip's world that Lindbergh is going to disenfranchise and demean Jewish Americans, just as Hitler is reported to be doing to Jewish Germans. The first indication of this policy is a plan to disperse Jewish children to rural areas. Philip's elder brother Sandy is packed off to a tobacco farm in Kentucky, where, to his father's disgust, he has a marvellous time. Philip's delinquent cousin Alvin, on the other hand, runs off to Canada where he enlists in the Army and loses a leg while fighting the Germans in France. Philip's maternal aunt marries the sinister Rabbi Bengelsdorf, who actually works for President Lindbergh, who he claims is no longer anti-Semitic and only wants the best for his Jewish American citizens. Meanwhile, Philip's parents struggle to keep their family afloat and remain fiercely loyal to Roosevelt's democratic ideals. Things go from bad to worse. There is violence and heartbreak, and you have to keep reminding yourself that none of this really happened. Eventually the nightmare history rejoins reality, but I'm not going to spoil your anticipation by telling you how this happens. Roth's account of childhood is written with masterly skill, and is a pleasure to read. It would have been good without the alternative history, but the nightmare scenario gives it an edgy, nervous excitement. Have you ever wondered what might happen if America elected the wrong president?

EVERYMAN (2006)

Now I want to slip Philip Roth's little black book into your hands. It will fit easily into your pocket, so you can carry it around and read it anywhere. It's called *Everyman*, and it's about death. On page one, the hero (known to us only as Everyman) is already dead, and we are present at his funeral. The mourners include the second (and most loved) of his three wives, his two sons, his daughter, his brother, and the nurse with whom he had an affair after his first bout of cardiac surgery. This is only the first of three visits to the old Jewish cemetery, so we shall get to know it quite well. When the funeral is over, we flash back to Everyman's childhood and go through his life story. He grows up in a small town in New Jersey, where his father owns a jewellery shop and teaches his son all about diamonds. As in previous novels, Roth describes the craftsmanship of the older generation with loving detail. When the boy grows up he becomes the art director of an advertising agency, but we don't hear much about his work. We do learn a lot about his marriages, his daughter Nancy whom he loves devotedly, and his infidelities. Disgracefully, he cheats on Nancy's mother by having an affair with a 24-year-old model. I am pleased to report that although this is a book about dying, the sex scenes are in the best Roth style. Although brief, they don't disappoint. And then there are the illnesses and the operations. As a child, our hero has to have a hernia repaired. He survives, but the boy in the next bed dies in the night – an early intimation of mortality. In his thirties, Everyman survives peritonitis from a missed appendix, and then remains well until he is 56, when the first heart attack strikes. After that it's a quintuple bypass and a series of angioplasties at intervals down the years to keep the blood flowing to his kidneys and brain as well as to his heart. When he retires at the age of 65, he decides to devote himself to painting, and gives art classes to the other residents of the Starfish Beach retirement colony. Throughout the latter part of his life his friends keep dying. As he reflects at one point, 'Old age isn't a battle; old age is a massacre.' As he moves inexorably closer to his own departure date, I am reminded of Tolstoy's classic novella *The Death of Ivan Ilyich*. And I guess Roth must have had it in mind as well. Both start with the death of the hero and proceed to reflect on his life. The difference is that whereas Ivan concludes that his life has been lived the wrong way, Everyman tells himself (and his readers) that there is no changing who you are: 'You just have to hold your ground and take it as it comes.' The ageing Philip Roth has lost none of his skills as a writer, and much of his little black book is very moving. I recommend the scene with the gravedigger (shades of Hamlet!) near the end, in which another craftsman's dedication is beautifully described. Yes, Everyman is back in the old cemetery visiting his parents, because he needs to talk with their bones. 'Your boy is seventy-one', he tells them, sadly. Their replies are reassuring. And the last paragraph is just beautiful. So please get a copy of *Everyman* and enjoy it. Then keep it by your bed.

KAZUO ISHIGURO was born in Nagasaki, Japan in 1954, and moved to England with his family at the age of six. He went to a boys' grammar school in Surrey and did a degree in English and Philosophy at the University of Kent. Like Ian McEwan, he enrolled for the MA in Creative Writing at the University of East Anglia. His first major success as a novelist was with *The Remains of the Day*, the memoirs of a devoted butler who worked in a stately home in the 1930s and found it difficult to get in touch with his emotions. This novel won the Booker Prize in 1989 and was later turned into a very successful film with Antony Hopkins and Emma Thompson in the leading roles. The next two novels, *When We Were Orphans* (2000) and *Never Let Me Go* (2005), were both shortlisted for the Booker Prize, and are reviewed here. Ishiguro writes in the first person and is a beautiful stylist. I am impatiently waiting for his next book to appear.

WHEN WE WERE ORPHANS (2000)

The hero of this Ishiguro novel is a detective. Not a policeman, as he is at pains to make clear, but a brilliant 'consultant' like Sherlock Holmes or Lord Peter Wimsey. Did such people ever exist in real life? It is hard to say, but Christopher Banks seems to be making quite a success of his profession, having solved several notoriously difficult 'cases' which have left Scotland Yard baffled. The book is set mainly in the 1920s and 1930s, and Ishiguro's prose has an aristocratic period elegance which is quite convincing.

Gradually we learn more about Christopher's childhood. He lived with his European parents in the British colony of Shanghai until the age of ten, when first his father and then his mother mysteriously disappeared. The other adults lead Christopher to believe that his parents have been kidnapped because of their opposition to the opium trade. He is hurriedly brought to England and slotted into the public school system, where he does his best to blend in. After a while we realise that he wants to become a private detective so that he can return to Shanghai and rescue his parents, whom he believes are still alive.

In England, Christopher mixes in upper-class society, solving crimes but also keeping an eye on developments in the East. He is attracted to other orphans, including a glamorous young woman called Sarah, and a little girl called Jennifer whom he decides to adopt. The story then flashes back to his boyhood in Shanghai and his friendship with a Japanese boy with whom he plays a game about looking for his father.

Eventually the grown up Christopher returns to Shanghai, and in the middle of the Sino-Japanese war he fights his way through shell-damaged houses, trying to find the house where he believes his parents are still held captive. This part of the book is very gripping, and you don't know whether to believe he will really find his parents or not. In the end there is a brutal disillusionment for Christopher as he learns some painful truths about his past. But his spirit, enclosed in a tough protective shell, is undefeated, and in a moving final chapter he achieves a kind of peace.

In family practice we can often understand our patients' problems better if we know something about their childhood and their experiences with their parents. Like Christopher, we may have to do some detective work to help our patients to trace the origin of their psychosomatic symptoms. *When We Were Orphans* made me think about how we seem to need the continued presence and unconditional love of our internal parents all the way to the end of our own lives.

NEVER LET ME GO (2005)

This is another subtly beautiful novel that will touch your heart and have you nervously checking your other organs. Kazuo Ishiguro has a very simple translucent style that is entirely English, and yet he gives me the impression that he might come from a different planet. *Never Let Me Go* has elements of the school story and of bioscience fiction. It seems to be about clones, but I suspect that it's really about what life has in store for all of us. Let me explain. The story is told in the first person by 31-year-old Kathy, who tells us that she is a 'carer', whose job is to look after 'donors.' Gradually we realise that when Kathy has finished being a carer she will become a donor herself. She and her friends are all clones who have been produced as living banks for spare organs. We are never told what organs are involved, but I suspect it starts with kidneys and goes on to parts that are less easy to do without. No one survives 'fourth donation', and some only manage two or three before they 'complete.' I think you can guess what that means.

The first part of the book is about the childhood of Kathy and her best friends, Ruth and Tommy. They go to a rather special school called Hailsham that reproduces many of the features of a first-class English public school. Here the teachers (called guardians) give them a good education and try to help them to live a life that will be as fulfilling as possible, despite its inevitable brevity. The school seems to care for them and gives them a sense of community, although of course they have no parents. Do they know that they are going to die in the operating theatre in their twenties or thirties? As Miss Lucy, one of the guardians, says, they are 'told and not told.' They know it will happen one day, but the details are not filled in.

A strange feature of the book is that we learn nothing about how the cloning programme developed and became accepted. There is no discussion of the ethical issues. The story is chiefly about the relationships of the three main characters, first at school and later in their adult world of donors and carers. At school, they confide in each other and become very close. They also have secrets and can be teasing and cruel, especially Ruth. She and Tommy become lovers in their last year at Hailsham, where sex is allowed, although not encouraged. Quite a lot of clones become couples. They know that they can never have children, but there is a rumour that couples who are really in love may be allowed a few extra years together before they have to start donating their organs. Another important activity at Hailsham is producing artwork, the best of which is taken away by the mysterious 'Madame' who visits the school regularly and is believed to display them in her Gallery. The children have a vague belief that it is important for everyone to be creative because their art will reveal that despite being clones, they are human beings with souls. Kathy and her friends never challenge the system that has so cynically given them life, only to harvest them for spare parts. They accept their ultimate fate, but they do struggle to find some meaning in their lives, and this is very moving. Although they are made and not born, perhaps the clone children are not really so different from the rest of us. Like them, we are given a life that can be sweet, but one day it will be taken away from us, probably before we are ready.

JOSÉ SARAMAGO was born in Portugal in 1922. He left school early and did a number of jobs, including manual work and journalism, before becoming a full-time writer. In 1969 he joined the Portuguese Communist Party, a brave step in the time of the fascist Salazar regime. A further clash with the authorities came with the publication of *The Gospel According to Jesus Christ* in 1991. In this novel (which I strongly recommend), Saramago gives an alterative version of the gospel story in which Jesus questions his role, argues with God, and is seen to be very human. The book was banned in Portugal, and Saramago emigrated to the Spanish island of Lanzarote. He was awarded the Nobel Prize for Literature in 1998.

BLINDNESS (1995)

Blindness is a gripping and very scary novel in which the people living in a city suddenly go blind, one after another, until nearly everyone is affected. The story starts with a group of cars waiting at a pedestrian crossing. When the lights go green, the lead car in the middle lane doesn't move. The driver has gone blind – all he can see is a uniform whiteness. Another man offers to drive him home, and the blind man gratefully accepts. Then the Good Samaritan steals his car, only to go blind himself a few blocks further on. The scene switches to an ophthalmologist's consulting room, where the first man has been brought, frantic for help. The doctor is puzzled as the history is unhelpful and examination reveals absolutely nothing wrong with the patient's eyes. Back at home, he starts to review the literature, but later that evening, yes, you've guessed it, he goes blind too, and as he ruefully says to himself, a blind ophthalmologist is not much good to anyone. More and more people succumb to the whiteout, and the only person to escape the plague is the doctor's wife. Prudently concealing the fact that she can still see, she becomes the heroine and saviour of the group of blind people in whose terrible adventures we are now compellingly caught up.

The authorities overreact with clumsy cruelty, and confine all the blind people in an empty mental hospital. They have decided that the blindness must be contagious, so the victims and those with whom they have come into contact must be isolated. Food is supplied, but the blind inmates of the ward have to come out and collect it themselves. The doors are guarded by soldiers who panic and shoot some of the victims who, in their anxiety and blindness, have approached too close. A group of blind criminals arrives and commandeers all the food, allowing meagre rations to the others only when they have surrendered all their valuables. Then they demand that all the blind women be handed over.

Yes, it's a nightmare world, but so vividly created that you have to keep turning the pages. And there are some acts of decency and kindness as well, showing that the better part of human nature can always survive, somewhere, somehow. Saramago has an interesting and unusual way of writing dialogue in this book. There are no quotation marks. Conversations may all take place in a single sentence, each person's speech starting with a capital letter and ending with a comma. Here is an example:

> He took me home, it's true, but then took advantage of my condition to steal my car, That's a lie, I didn't steal anything, You most certainly did, If anyone nicked your car it wasn't me, my reward for carrying out a kind action was to lose my sight.

Once you get used it, this style draws you powerfully into the conversation. Perhaps this kind of continuous flow is what speech sounds like when you can't see anyone.

If you are put off by the thought of a tale in which things go rapidly from bad to obscenely horrible, I must assure you that the book has a happy ending. On the last page, the doctor wonders why they all went blind, and his wife says:

> I don't think we did go blind, I think we are blind, Blind but seeing, Blind people who can see but don't see.

What they (and we) too often fail to see is amply described in this amazing book.

THE YEAR OF THE DEATH OF RICARDO REIS (1984)

Last summer I visited the beautiful city of Lisbon. I had never been there before, but in my imagination I had already been wandering through the steep streets and delightful squares of the old city with the help of Saramago's novel, *The Year of the Death of Ricardo Reis*. When the story opens, the year is 1935, and Dr Reis (who by the way is a GP and a poet) has just arrived in Lisbon by sea after a 16-year stay in Brazil. After checking into a hotel (giving us the pleasure of reading some wonderful descriptions of hotel life), he revisits some of his old haunts in the city. He goes to the cemetery to see the grave of the great Portuguese poet Fernando Pessoa, who has recently died. Now things begin to get a little uncanny. The dead Pessoa starts coming back to visit Ricardo in his hotel room. We learn that 'Ricardo Reis' is actually a fictitious character invented by Pessoa as one of a number of alter egos. And yet he is as real as you could wish, with his own engaging personality. He takes us around Lisbon, observing the people with an ironic yet compassion-ate eye, reflecting on life and death, politics and philosophy, and quoting lines of his own poetry. *I am astonished that you have said nothing about the women he loves.* Please Dorothy, I was just coming to that. *Well, I don't think I can trust you. I had better take over at this point. You see, ladies and gentlemen, Dr Reis is a man who loves women, and women love him. First, there is Lydia, who is a cleaner in the Hotel Bragança. When she brings the doctor his breakfast he holds on to her arm and something sexy sparks bet-ween them. That evening she arranges his bed so that there are two pillows side by side! Of course she visits him in the night and they become lovers. But there is another woman! The sad, beautiful Marcenda stays in the hotel with her father, the lawyer. Marcenda has a paralysed left arm that she holds in her right hand like a wounded bird. Ricardo encourages her to reveal the psychosomatic origins of her paralysis. You doctors will like this very much because he is so clever and yet so sympathetic. Of course he falls in love with her, too.* Please Dorothy. *All right, I have finished now, but thanks to me they will want to read the book that you made sound* so *boring.* Well, I don't think that's fair, but I will just finish by telling you that if you go to the delightful Café Brasilia in Lisbon's Chiado district, you will find a life-size bronze figure of Fernando Pessoa, seated at one of the outside tables just waiting to have a chat with you about life and literature. And, of course, love. *That's better.*

SEBASTIAN FAULKS was born in Newbury, Berkshire in 1953. He was the first literary editor of *The Independent* newspaper, and later became its dep-uty editor. His first novel, *A Trick of the Light*, was published in 1984. He went on to write three novels about love, war and France, which were his principal subjects in the 1990s. *Birdsong* (1993) is about the experiences of a young Englishman in the First World War, *Charlotte Grey* (1998) is about the French resistance movement in the Second World War, and *On Green Dolphin Street* (2001) deals with the Cold War period in the 1950s. More recently, as we shall see in the two books reviewed below, Faulks seems to have become interested in psychiatry and the disturbing instability of the human mind. In 1998, he took some time off from serious literature to produce the latest James Bond novel (*Devil May Care*), which I'm told is very good if you like that sort of thing.

HUMAN TRACES (2005)

This one is a really nice long read. It's a broad, sweeping, panoramic novel with lots of medical interest. It tells the story of two young men, one French and one English, who both grow up in the last quarter of the nineteenth century with a compelling ambition to understand the nature of mental illness.

The French boy, Jacques, lives in rural Brittany and has an older brother, Olivier, who has had to be banished to the stables because of his weird talk and strange behaviour. He is clearly schizophrenic, although the word has not yet been invented. Meanwhile, Thomas Midwinter, a merchant's son who lives in England, is encouraged by his sister to become a medical student, although his main interest is in literature. Faulks brings his two young heroes together when Thomas takes a holiday in France (I forgive him for this device, because by now I am involved in the story, and the sooner the two boys meet up the better). While they both have equal enthusiasm for the subject of madness, their approaches are contrasted. Thomas is fascinated by Mr Darwin's book and wonders how human madness survived natural selection. He also feels that the answers will lie embedded in the structure of the brain. Jacques, on the other hand, is driven by the emotional pressure to somehow rescue his beloved brother whose life has been wasted by his illness.

As the two boys pursue their separate studies, we are allowed to witness the early stages of psychiatric history. We eavesdrop on the legendary Professor Charcot demonstrating the physical basis of hysteria in the Salpêtrière clinic in Paris. Back in England we are plunged into a nightmarish Victorian asylum (not very different from the ones I visited as a student), where thousands of desperate, undiagnosed patients crowd round young Thomas clamouring for attention. Eventually the two young mad-doctors set up a clinic together in an old castle in the Austrian Alps, where they combine practice and research. You may be wondering when Sigmund Freud is going to make an appearance. Strangely, he is never mentioned by name, although there are oblique references to the 'Vienna School.' However, Jacques begins treating an attractive young woman with apparently hysterical symptoms by a method that looks suspiciously like psychoanalysis. Thomas reads the case notes and is horrified – it seems clear to him that her abdominal pain is due to torsion of an ovarian cyst. This leads to coolness between the two heroes, their theoretical orientations diverge, and their friendship is never quite the same. I should add that the book is as much about the lives and emotions of its characters as it is about the history of psychiatry. Jacques marries Thomas's sister, and Thomas falls in love with Jacques' 'hysterical' patient. There are brilliantly written diversionary episodes in central Africa (Thomas tracing the origins of man) and the battlefields of the First World War. I really enjoyed *Human Traces*, which was recommended to me by my friend Leon, who is a psychiatrist. Although he is not a great novel reader, he was enthralled by this one. I am left pondering the book's most intriguing idea, which is Thomas's theory that the human vulnerability to madness is the price we pay for the development of our unique brain. The amazingly complex cerebral cortex allows us to be conscious and know who we are, but there's a serious risk of our thoughts and memories slipping out of control.

ENGLEBY (2007)

Although I'm quite a sociable person (as Dorothy will confirm), I like a story about a loner, in which he tells his own story and reveals his secret thoughts, as if to a diary. *The Curious Incident of the Dog in the Night-Time* is a memorable example. Most literary loners are a little strange, but telling your own confidential story is a good way to enlist the reader's sympathy. However, a word of warning is necessary. The narrative may be unreliable, and the friendly voice that whispers in your ear may turn out to have a serious personality disorder.

This is the case with Mike Engleby, the narrator and chief subject (I nearly said suspect) of *Engleby*. Mike introduces himself as a student at an ancient university (fairly clearly Cambridge). He has a fine sense of irony, and his satirical account of university life in the 1970s is very entertaining. But we can't help noticing that he has no real friends, he drinks rather a lot, he uses of a lot of cannabis and he takes a little blue ten-milligram pill every night. He also steals from shops and from people's clothes. He is very interested in a fellow student called Jennifer, but there is not much hope of a normal healthy boy-and-girl relationship here. Mike follows Jennifer around timidly and tries to imagine her life with her friends. He is obsessed with her, but we later realise from some extracts from her diary (which Mike has stolen) that she is only dimly aware of him as an odd bloke who keeps cropping up everywhere.

How did Mike, with his wit and intelligence, get to be such a sad, lonely, obsessive boy? We learn that his childhood was bleak and that his asthmatic father used to beat him. At public school he was bullied systematically (horrific reading) and became a bully himself. University life might have liberated him, and we retain a shred of hope until Jennifer mysteriously disappears. Mike knows more about this than he lets on even to himself. I don't know how much more I should tell you. I'll just say that there are some police

CHAPTER 5

A handful of classic novels

There used to be an excellent second-hand bookshop next door to the Green Bookshop, but sadly it had to close because the lease expired. All of the classics were available there, some of them in excellent condition and all reasonably priced. To fill the gap, we decided to open our own Classics Corner, a comfortable enclave where you can immerse yourself in the literary masterpieces of the past.

The Green Bookshop is very keen on the classics. They have been around a long time and have proved their worth. They are good. They are reliable. Furthermore, they can be read many times and always yield something new that you didn't notice before.

If you read a classic when you are young and then again in middle age, it will reveal something different to you the second time, because you are no longer quite the same person.

ANNA KARENINA by Leo Tolstoy (1876)

So pour yourself a coffee and follow me please to Classics Corner, where I want to show you one of the greatest of all stories, and one of my special favourites. I keep it on my bedside table so that I can open it at random and read a chapter or two before I go to sleep. It is of course Tolstoy's wonderful *Anna Karenina*. If you have read it before, it's almost certainly time to read it again. If you haven't, then prepare yourself for an eye-opening, inner-life-enhancing literary treat. If you find thick nineteenth-century novels intimidating, don't worry. The great thing about Tolstoy is that he is *really easy to read*. His characters spring immediately to life, and he has this magical ability to make you feel that you are there beside them, sharing their lives. You almost certainly know about the beautiful Anna and her passionate adulterous love affair with the handsome officer, Count Vronsky. But Tolstoy entwines with their story another one about a couple, Levin and Kitty, whose lives are more like our own. Levin, when we meet him, is a young man up from the country who feels very awkward in sophisticated Moscow society. But he is determined to find and propose to 18-year-old Kitty, with whom he is seriously in love. There is a wonderful chapter in which he meets her, as if by chance, at the skating rink (a fashionable place to hang out) and they skim round the ice together. But then his hopes are dashed because Kitty has fallen for Vronsky, who of course will forget all about her as soon as he catches sight of Anna with that beautiful dark hair curling over her shoulders . . . You see how easily I get carried away, and you will be, too, I promise. I don't want to reveal too much of the story, but I will tell you that while Anna and Vronsky's affair ends in tragedy, Levin and Kitty eventually do get married and live happily despite his tendency to worry about the meaning of life. Fortunately, Kitty is very wise and practical as well as pretty. And you will also meet Anna's unreliable but very sympathetic brother Steve, who is married to Kitty's elder sister, Dolly. In fact the story starts with Steve trying to rescue his marriage after Dolly has found out about his affair with the French governess. Soon you will feel that you know all these people intimately and be very concerned about them. Tolstoy has a unique gift of making your heart beat in sympathy with all his characters, including even Anna's rather obnoxious husband. So here, let me present you with a copy. It's a new translation which they tell me is very good, although I prefer to stick to the one by Rosemary Edmonds that I first read all those years ago in my teens.

* * * * *

I was just idly re-arranging the Jane Austen section when I became aware of two young ladies in long gowns of sprigged muslin peering at me through the glass pane in the door. The latch clicked, the bell tinkled softly, and they came in arm in arm and smiling sweetly.

'Good afternoon, sir' said one of them. 'My friend and I would be most obliged if you could show us some new books, for we are both excessively fond of reading.'

'It will be a pleasure, ladies,' I replied. 'Do you care for history? We have some excellent new historical books.' 'I detest history!' said her friend with a shudder. 'The men all so good for nothing and hardly any women at all – it is very tiresome. Have you no Radcliffe books?' 'We have many,' I replied, 'but they are mostly of a medical nature and not suitable for young ladies.' 'No, no, I mean books by Mrs Anne Radcliffe, the lady novelist. Did you never read her *Mysteries of Udolpho*? It is a most delightful and horrid tale. My brother finished it in two days, his hair standing on end throughout.'

'Now I understand', I said with a deep bow, 'and I think I may have just the thing . . .'

NORTHANGER ABBEY by Jane Austen (1818)

It's called *Northanger Abbey* and it was one of the first of Jane Austen's major works to be written, although it was not published until after her death. Although it is in typical Jane Austen style, it's also quite unusual because its subtext is all about writers and readers. There are lots of jokes about the novels of the day and their impressionable readers. She even gives us a running commentary on how to write a best-seller (with tongue in cheek, of course).

Now for the story. Our heroine is a girl called Catherine Morley who is only 17, so this is almost a book for teenagers. Jane Austen tells us that she has been 'training for a heroine' since the age of 15, because she and her friends are all avid novel readers. At the time the most popular novels were 'sentimental' – that is, either very soppy and emotional, or 'Gothic', in which case they added frightening elements such as ghosts, ruined castles, murder and mystery. When Catherine is invited by witty, charming Henry Tilney to stay at his family's ruined abbey, she is thrilled to bits and looks forward to a really frightening time. In her bedroom there is a mysterious black cabinet. What can it contain? That night, as a furious storm rages outside, she opens the drawers and finds an ancient document. What can it be? Before she can read it, the wind blows out her candle and she spends the whole night in delicious terror. However, in the morning the document proves to be only an old laundry list. Then there is Henry's father, the moody General Tilney, who is every inch the typical villain of Gothic fiction. Catherine is convinced that he must have murdered his late wife or, at the very least, locked her up in a secret room in the abbey.

You will be glad to hear that, as well as having all these fantasies, Catherine is given the sort of romantic plot that a true heroine deserves. The girl she thought was her best friend turns out to be a heartless schemer, and her brother is even worse. She finds true love with young Henry, but their future is almost blighted by the General, who has been deceived into thinking that her parents have no money. In truth, they are not super-rich but not completely broke either. Catherine is dismissed from the house, and believes that they all hate her. She suffers real pain, as Jane Austen shows us how a world-class novelist can create characters we really care about. Then she wraps the whole thing up with a happy ending, rather like Mozart concluding a heart-stopping opera with a cheerful little ensemble. Wonderful. Our young friends have taken a copy each.

*   *   *   *   *

It was a gloomy November morning in the High Street, but the sun was doing his best to pierce the clouds with his cheerfully illuminating rays. And on this particular November morning the proprietor of the Green Bookshop, that noble emporium of the printed word and supplier of reading pleasure to the quality and gentry, having opened his shutters and flung open the door to greet his customers, was apprised of an unusual sight. Standing on the door-step was a short, stout gentleman, with a large bald cranium, whose bright eyes twinkled beneficently from behind a pair of small round spectacles. His attire, although well tailored, was strikingly antique in style. His white shirt was finished at the neck with a flowing stock and covered by a black waist-coat. Over this he wore a bright blue tailcoat, and the ensemble was completed in the nether regions by tights, gaiters and buckled shoes.

'Good day, sir' said the Antique Gentleman, 'could you tell me if the mail coach to Bath leaves from these premises?'

'It does not, my friend,' replied the proprietor, 'for this is a bookshop, but if you will walk a little way down Cheapside you will come to an inn called the George and Vulture, from which coaches depart four times daily.'

I beg your pardon?

Oh hello there. Do excuse me, I must have been having a nap and I thought you were Mr Pickwick. Yes, that's right, Dickens. I've just finished reading **THE PICKWICK PAPERS** (1837), and the characters are all in my head. Do you like Dickens? You're not sure? Well, yes, he is a bit long, but what's the hurry? Let me tell you about Pickwick, which is a really good one to start with. It's one of his first, it's stuffed with wonderful characters, many of whom you will find you know already, and it's incredibly funny.

What is it about? Well, Mr Pickwick is a plump amiable gentleman (founder of the Pickwick Club) who decides to take three younger friends on a series of coach journeys round the South of England in search of what you might describe as interesting encounters and experiences. The three friends are Mr Tracy Tupman (an ageing Romeo), Mr Augustus Snodgrass (an aspiring poet) and Mr Nathaniel Winkle (an inept sportsman). And what adventures they have! They are involved in courtships, seductions, weddings, duels, a rural cricket match and a scandalously corrupt by-election.

They fall victim to the shabby, genteel conman Mr Alfred Jingle, taken in by his attractively hesitant staccato speech, punctuated with dashes. Here, by way of illustration, is one of Jingle's most famous tall stories, related to a credulous Mr Pickwick as their coach passes under a low arch:

> Terrible place – dangerous work – other day – five children – mother – tall lady eating sandwiches – forgot the arch – crash – knock – children look round – mother's head off – sandwich in hand – no mouth to put it in – head of a family off – shocking, shocking.

The Pickwicks are also befriended by the generous Mr Wardle, a country gentleman and resident of the delightfully named village of Dingley Dell. We get to meet his large family, which includes two nubile daughters and a romantically inclined spinster aunt. The household also contains Joe, a fat boy with sleep apnoea ('Joe! – damn that boy, he's gone to sleep again.') Gentle, chivalrous Mr Pickwick accidentally delivers what sounds like a marriage proposal to his landlady, Mrs Bardell, as a result of which she is encouraged to sue him by the rascally lawyers Dodson and Fogg (we all know them). When he refuses to pay damages, he is consigned to the Fleet Prison, where he acquits himself with honour and dignity.

And of course Mr Pickwick engages as his manservant and protector, Mr Sam Weller, the man who mixes up his Vs and his Ws as many cockneys used to do. Sam is efficient, street-wise and totally imperturbable, and can handle anyone, whatever their social position. He and his governor are a classic master–servant pair, like Don Quixote and Sancho Panza, or Bertie Wooster and Jeeves. I could go on – but I can't tell it the way Dickens does. His descriptive style may seem long-winded, but it's full of delicious irony, and the many conversations in Pickwick are crackling with life and energy.

NORTH AND SOUTH by Elizabeth Gaskell (1846)

Now what have we here? A nice, thick, juicy Victorian novel called *North and South* by Elizabeth Gaskell. Charlotte Brontë you know, of course, but you may not have read anything by her friend and biographer, who is often rather patronisingly called 'Mrs Gaskell.' Elizabeth was a considerable novelist herself, although she doesn't have quite the same passion and fervour as Charlotte. What she does have, to a greater extent, is the ability to connect her characters with the wider world of which they are part. In *North and South* she starts off with a typical Victorian heroine, Margaret Hale, who is calmly observing the wedding preparations of her wealthier cousin and wondering what sort of wedding she would like for herself. But some shocks are in store. In chapter four, Margaret's life is turned upside down when her father, a country vicar, announces that he must give up his living because he can no longer subscribe to the rules of the Church of England as laid down in the Act of Uniformity, into the details of which we will not go just now. Instead he is going to drag Margaret and her mother off to an industrial manufacturing town called Milton (also known as Manchester) in the gloomy, filthy, clamorous, working-class north. Here she meets a handsome young mill owner called John Thornton who attempts to deal with some of her prejudices about manufacturing and trade. But there is trouble at the Thornton mill, and the striking workers besiege the factory. In the key scene of the novel, Margaret protects Thornton from the fury of the mob by throwing her arms around his neck and shielding him from the hail of stones and clogs that his employees are hurling at him. After this high drama and suppressed sexual passion there are, of course, many ups and downs, and I have to say that the pace flags a bit in the last 100 pages. But eventually the middle-class Margaret and her self-made capitalist are lovingly reunited. *North and South* was first published as a serial in Charles Dickens's weekly magazine 'Household Words.' Dickens had earlier published *Hard Times*, his own novel of life in the industrial north, in the same journal. Oh, and while I'm on the subject, David Lodge's *Nice Work* (2001) is a kind of parody of *North and South* in which a female English lecturer interacts with a male steelworks manager in the imaginary Midlands city of Rummidge. But read *North and South* first to appreciate all the jokes, especially the one about the 'knobstick.' I shall say no more.

THE TRIAL by Franz Kafka (written in 1914, published in 1925)

This begins with the famous chilling sentence 'Someone must have been telling lies about Joseph K, for without having done anything wrong he was arrested one fine morning.' But this is not the kind of arrest favoured by Joseph Stalin. For one thing, the suspect is not taken into custody, but encouraged to go to his job at the bank as usual. The arresting officers also behave very strangely.

They won't tell K what he is accused of, they eat his breakfast, and they offer to sell his clothes for him. At his first interrogation by the examining magistrate, K is heroically defiant and treats the whole weird legal apparatus with withering contempt. Then his uncle urges him to regard his predicament more seriously, and takes him along to meet a famous defence lawyer. Although the great man proves to be on his sickbed, he already knows about Joseph's case, which he finds very interesting. With lawyers, as with doctors, it is always an advantage to be 'an interesting case.' But Joseph, instead of being grateful, is easily distracted by the lawyer's nurse, who persuades him to slip into the next room with her for a hot date. There is a good deal of farcical humour in *The Trial*, and also a lot of casual sex, so you can see that reading it will not be the remorselessly grim experience you were expecting. When Joseph starts to find out more about how the courts operate, we are introduced to a legal system that seems totally bizarre and corrupt and at the same time strangely familiar.

Everything a lawyer says is immediately followed by its contradiction. The defendant's first written plea is of crucial importance, but it frequently gets lost, so that no one ever reads it. It is vital to have a good lawyer, but defending counsel are not allowed into the court and can only help their clients by chatting up the judges in private. Towards the end of the book, Joseph K has an interview with a priest in the cathedral, who tells him an enigmatic story about a man from the country who seeks 'admittance to the Law' from a bearded doorkeeper who bars his way. He is never allowed in although, when it is too late, he is told that 'this door was meant only for you.' This is one of Kafka's most famous and most inscrutable parables. The Law (with a capital L) now takes on a religious quality, and Joseph's unnamed crime is more like some sort of original sin for which he needs to seek absolution. Scholars and critics continue to argue about what Kafka means by the Law, and whether he really believed in God or not. No one really knows, and perhaps he didn't know himself. *The Trial* is full of mysteries (we are not even sure that the chapters are in the right order), but Kafka has a beautiful, lucid style and the book is easy to read. It will make you think and it will make you laugh.

American classics

One thing I love about American writers is that they all have such individual voices, which make them instantly recognisable and believable. It all started with Mark Twain, who lets Huckleberry Finn speak for himself in an American vernacular that no one had seen in print before. Then there is that tough guy, Ernest Hemingway – no mistaking him whether you like him or not. And there's another literary giant who you may not have gotten around to, by the name of William Faulkner. Like Mark Twain he was a Southerner who set his novels in rural Mississippi in the 1920s. Here's a novel I'd like to recommend, called *A Light in August*. It begins with a young country girl called Lena who has walked all the way from her home in Alabama to some-where in Mississippi ('a fur piece' as she puts it), and is hoping to hitch a lift into the town of Jefferson. Lena is heavily pregnant and has come in search of her baby's father. Our hearts sink when we hear that he 'had to go away' and promised to send for her but left no address. Nevertheless, Lena is ever hopeful of finding him, and I'm glad to say that people are helpful. After a few chapters, other characters start to creep into the story. There is an eccentric ex-minister called the Reverend Hightower, who has been dismissed by his congregation for various reasons, including his wife's scandalous behaviour and his crazy sermons. Then there is the tragic and mysterious Joe Christmas, who folks say is part Negro, although no one really knows. Where did he come from? Is it true that he is selling illicit whisky, and just what is his rela-tionship with that Miss Burden who lives by herself and is known to visit with black families in the neighbourhood?

Faulkner is like a brilliant storyteller sitting in his chair with his audience gathered round him. He does the voices of the country people, but he also has a narrator's voice, which is rich, poetical and sometimes biblical. The narrat-ive jumps about in time, sometimes giving us a character's background long after we think we know all that there is to know about him. After a while you almost feel that you live in that little town with its poverty, lack of edu-cation, racial prejudice and long memories of the Civil War and slavery. At times you wonder whether Mr Faulkner is telling the story or dreaming it. I have to warn you that terrible things happen, but there is a hopeful ending, and Lena and her baby emerge OK.

Like many American writers, Faulkner spent some time as a screenwriter in Hollywood, where he had mixed fortunes. He adapted Raymond Chandler's thriller *The Big Sleep*, which became a classic film noir starring Humphrey Bogart and Lauren Bacall (*see* Chapter 7 on books and the cinema, or better still, see the film). Just a little way along the shelf from Faulkner, but still in the F section, we come to his contemporary, Scott Fitzgerald, who also did a stint in Hollywood. Fitzgerald was brilliantly talented, but unhappily drank himself to death at the age of 44. He wrote one perfect book called *The Great Gatsby*, which is a joy to read, despite its tragic subject of an American Dream that is abruptly terminated. Unlike Faulkner, Fitzgerald was fascinated by rich and successful people, and he loved to party with them. You must treat yourself to Gatsby (it's very short – you can read it in an evening and then read it again). But I would also like to recommend his final, unfinished novel called *The Last Tycoon*. This is a thing of shreds and patches, but it has one terrific chapter about a day in the life of a movie mogul and supervisor of productions called Monroe Stahr. The character of Stahr was closely modelled on the legendary Irving Thalberg, who worked for Louis B Mayer at MGM until his premature death in 1932. Thalberg (known as 'The Boy Wonder') was not just a money man – he had culture and taste, and he cared deeply about the content and style of the films that he had to churn out endlessly. The book offers a glimpse inside a studio in Hollywood's golden age as captured by another boy wonder with not much longer to live.

An Indian classic: *MIDNIGHT'S CHILDREN* by Salman Rushdie (1981)

Midnight's Children won the Booker Prize for Salman Rushdie in 1981, and was subsequently honoured twice more by the Booker judges. On different occasions in the last few years, it was voted the Book of Bookers and the Best of Bookers. As it has been around for nearly 30 years, we have decided that it has earned its place as a modern classic.

Now I have a confession to make. Sitting on my bookshelf at home is the hardback copy of *Midnight's Children* that I bought in 1981. I had several goes at reading it, but never managed to get beyond the second chapter. I seemed to be immune to the charms of Rushdie's playfully idiosyncratic prose style. I just wasn't ready, you see. Because when I started it again earlier this year I was like a duck in a pond. I just paddled around happily, gulping deep mouthfuls. So my advice is, if you are not ready for a book that is clearly a great one, just put it aside for a decade or two and then try again. The result will be magic.

How can I tell you about *Midnight's Children*? It's the life story of a young man called Saleem Sinai who was born along with 1000 other Indian babies between midnight and 1 am on the day that India became independent (15 August 1947).

He is telling his story to a woman called Padma, with whom he is evidently on intimate terms. She manages a pickle and chutney factory, and while Saleem tells his story she stirs a vast vat of pickle mixture and interjects impatiently, trying to get him to keep to the point. The story takes a long time to tell (there are many convolutions and digressions, as in its eighteenth-century predecessor, *Tristram Shandy*), and the set-up also comically resembles the *Thousand and One Nights* of Scheherazade. Salman Rushdie has described his book as a biography of India – a tragedy told as a comedy.

It's fascinating to compare it with *The White Tiger*, winner of the 2008 Man Booker Prize (*see* Chapter 2). Rushdie was obviously a major influence on Aravind Adiga, but his style is very different and much more elaborate. You will either love it or hate it.

The first page and a bit (the preamble) provide a good sample:

> I was born at midnight . . . once upon a time. No, that won't do, there's no get-ting away from the date: I was born in Dr Narlikar's nursing home on August 15th 1947. And the time? The time matters, too.

You will notice lots of hesitations, and rephrasing as if Saleem is shuffling ideas in his mind. Then he will come up with a series of stunning metaphors:

> On the stroke of midnight as a matter of fact. Clock hands joined in respectful greeting as I came . . . Thanks to the occult tyrannies of those blandly saluting clocks I had been mysteriously handcuffed to history, my destinies chained to those of my country.

Soon Saleem is carried away on a great tide of enthusiastic grandiloquence: 'I have been a swallower of lives. Consumed multitudes are jostling and shoving inside me' (shades of Walt Whitman!). Then he hints at mysterious happenings that will have incalculable consequences ('the memory of a large white bedsheet with a roughly circular hole some seven inches in diameter cut in the centre'). And the sheet is stained with 'three drops of old faded redness.' All this will be explained in good time, if we are patient. The style is always playful, but we are constantly reminded that the story of the birth and child-hood of independent India (and Pakistan) is a tragedy.

We have to wait a few chapters before Saleem gets himself born. But the tale of his grandfather the doctor, his beguiling patient and that holey bed sheet will keep you happy while you wait. Saleem describes himself as an unat-tractive baby. He has a moon face, stains on his cheeks, prominences on his temples and a nose the size and shape of a cucumber. During his childhood and adolescence he undergoes a series of accidents, each of which confers strange powers on him which will profoundly affect his destiny and that of India. He hides in a washing chest and, while peeping out, sees his mother's naked bottom as she undresses for her lover. He gives an almighty sniff and finds that he is hearing voices! These prove to be the voices of all the other surviving children born in India in the first hour of independence. They all have gifts, some supernatural, and they are able to talk to each other through Saleem's mediation, like a huge parliament. If you think this is bizarre, it's called Magical Realism and it's the fictional trope of presenting magical events as if there was no need to explain them. They just happen and are accepted. Saleem hopes that the Children of Midnight will somehow act as a moderating force, in favour of peace and reason despite all of the inter-ethnic violence that is erupting after independence. But it is not to be. There are wars with the Chinese, with Pakistan, and between Pakistan's two wings, with India supporting Bangladesh. Thousands are killed, including, it seems, most of Saleem's many relatives. And so he ends up telling the story to Padma in the pickle factory and, if and when you get to the end, your sadness will be mitigated by the news that Saleem has agreed to marry his Padma. You will also have enjoyed a wonderful tragicomic saga full of literary splendour. Dorothy, what did you think? Did you read it in 1981?

Do you mind? I was still at school in 1981 and the nuns wouldn't let us read that kind of thing. But I did get to it later and I loved it. Having read it again I think I got more out of it the second time. Of course there are lots more women you didn't mention – that old Rushdie and his women! There's Saleem's sister (with whom he falls in love) and Parmati-the-Witch and behind them all, the menacing figure of 'The Widow' – Indira Gandhi herself, India's cruel mother. Wow! Dorothy, you are sending shivers down my spine! Listen, folks, if you don't have a first edition tucked away at home somewhere, we have lots of paperback copies for you to take away and read. Now or in a few years' time.

CHAPTER 6

Short stories and essays

Let's start with short stories, and later on we'll segue into essays, which I hope to persuade you are almost the same thing.

This week the Green Bookshop is holding a special Short Story Festival. Dorothy and I have been busy clearing space, ordering books, designing posters and putting short story displays in the window. Why short stories? Well, they are often neglected because people feel that they need some big piece of fiction to get their teeth into. There is also a tendency to feel a little bit cheated by a short story because, just as you are getting to know the characters and taking a keen interest in their future, the whole thing is suddenly over and you have to start again.

But the best short stories can do something special. They deliver a powerful emotional charge which is all the more effective because it is so compressed. A great short story can leave you feeling amused, excited, shocked, disturbed or moved to tears. Some stories have a twist in the tail, while others come to a gentle close but suggest that the main characters have undergone a moment of self-discovery that is going to change their lives.

So what sort of stories would you like to read? We shall be offering you a selection of the world's best, both singly and in collections. As you move through the display area you will find classic short stories from the nineteenth and twentieth centuries.

Let's start with some of the Russian masters of the nineteenth century. Tolstoy (1828–1910) wrote some great short stories as well as his major novels. *The Death of Ivan Ilyich* (a long short story) should be required reading for all doctors. It will help them to think about palliative care, and might also lead them on to *Anna Karenina*. Another marvellous Tolstoy tale is *Master and Man*, which recounts what happens when you and your servant embark on an ordinary sledge journey in the middle of the Russian winter, realise that you are lost, and then wonder if you are going to survive. Just next to Tolstoy we have his younger contemporary, Anton Chekhov (1860–1904). I am sure you know that Chekhov was a doctor, and we have every reason to glow with vicarious pride when we think of what our colleague has achieved. There is evidence that he was a very concerned and compassionate physician who treated poor people for nothing. He was also very affected by the conditions in the Siberian prison island of Sakhalin, about which he wrote a detailed report. Chekhov moved the short story into new territory by showing how effectively he could write about the comedy and tragedy of everyday lives. As his English translator David Magarshack says, 'On reading these stories one gets the impression of holding life itself, like a fluttering bird in one's cupped hands.'

May I suggest that you take home the Penguin collection *The Lady with the Little Dog*. The title story, one of Chekhov's most famous short stories, tells how a 40-year-old businessman and a younger woman (both married) embark on a casual affair and then find themselves deeply and painfully in love.

Next, I want to introduce another contender for the Green Bookshop Award for Best Short Story Ever Written. This one is by James Joyce. It is called 'The Dead' (don't be put off), and it's the last story of a collection called *Dubliners*, which he published in 1914. All of the stories are good, but 'The Dead' is special – it was even made into a very good film by John Huston. We start off at a grand Christmas Party in turn-of-the-century Dublin (wonderfully described), and finish with one of those heart-stopping moments of realisation that Joyce called 'epiphanies.' And it's so beautifully written. 'Snow was general all over Ireland . . . falling faintly through the universe and faintly falling like the descent of their last end, upon all the living and the dead.' You may have noticed that a lot of great short stories seem to have snow. For instance, in Kafka's 'A Country Doctor', a luckless GP has to drive through a blizzard to visit a patient in the next village. Is it just another unnecessary house call? Perhaps, but the horses are magic, the patient is not quite what he seems, and the practice will never be the same again. I shall not say any more about the Kafka stories just now, because we are going to meet him later on.

Now let's move on to the USA, which has had a special place in its heart for the short story ever since Edgar Allan Poe defined its particular qualities in 1842. He praised its singleness of purpose, and declared that the well-constructed short story would leave the reader with 'a sense of the fullest satisfaction.' American stories are full of juice and vigour, and they tell us a lot about the country and its people. Stephen Crane (who died at the age of 29) wrote about the Wild West and the senseless violence of frontier life. His story 'The Blue Hotel' is terrible in its inevitability. Flannery O'Connor casts a non-judgmental eye on the desperate, poverty-stricken and deeply prejudiced folk of the Deep South. I would recommend her story 'The Displaced Person.' If you prefer reading about more sophisticated city folk, you should go for Scott Fitzgerald. His classic story 'Bernice Bobs her Hair' tells of a depressed young girl's quest for social success, and has a riotously upbeat ending. Some of these stories might be difficult to find. I read them in an old book called *The American Short Story: Volume 1* (1977), collected and edited by Calvin Skaggs. I think it's probably out of print, but there are plenty of other collections available in which you can hunt for my favourites and enjoy lots of others. Oh yes, I mustn't forget Big Daddy himself, Ernest Hemingway, to whom so many modern short story writers acknowledge a debt. His deceptively simple prose style can be savoured in *The First Forty-Nine Stories*, which we do have in stock. Don't miss the story 'Indian Camp', which tells of a doctor who performs a Caesarean on a Native American woman without an anaesthetic: 'But her screams are not important. I don't hear them because they are not important.' Finally, let me mention a contemporary master, John Updike, who has been writing brilliant short stories about married life (and many other things) for 50 years. Updike is witty and perceptive and has a prose style that is full of delights. We have a fat and very satisfying collection of his stories right here on the shelf by your elbow.

* * * * *

If you share my belief in the important links between medicine and literature, you will want to take home a copy of *Doctors and Patients: an Anthology*. This is a collection of medical stories, both real-life and fictional, edited and introduced by Cecil Helman. The book is an intriguing mixture of different kinds of writing by all sorts of people. Famous literary doctor writers are represented by Anton Chekhov, William Carlos Williams, Arthur Conan Doyle, AJ Cronin, Mikhail Bulgakov and William Somerset Maugham. Some of the doctors portrayed are not very patient centred, I'm afraid, but that is probably part of the take-home message. Several of the patients' stories are true reports of their own experiences and these can be very moving.

With any anthology, you are bound to like some inclusions better than others. It's like listening to *Desert Island Discs* – you wonder 'Why on earth did he put that in? And why isn't there any Mozart/Bob Dylan?' My favourites among Cecil's selection would include Ruth Picardie's heartbreaking thoughts about dying too young, and Clive Sinclair's brilliantly satirical and metaphorical dispatch from the dialysis unit. I was gripped by Mikhail Bulgakov's terrified but triumphant obstetric performance, and it is always a pleasure to read anything by Oliver Sacks. I should add that Cecil has written a very nice and thought-provoking introductory essay, drawing on his resources as doctor, writer and anthropologist.

* * * * *

I was just closing up for the night and drawing the bolt across the door when I became aware of someone peering at me through the window. He was a tall, thin, wiry young fellow, wearing a smart suit and looking very anxious. Well, it was late, but I never like to turn away a customer, so I opened the door a crack and said 'Can I help you?' 'I think I am beyond help,' said he, with a smile, 'but I do need something to read.' 'Then this door was meant only for you,' I said. 'And I was just about to lock it.'

He looked a bit startled at that, so I let him in and he stood there, twitching and grimacing.

'What sort of books do you like?' I asked him. 'I think,' he said, 'we ought to read only the kind of books that wound and stab us. A book must be the axe for the frozen sea inside us.'

'I see,' I said. 'That was rather well put (which it was). You obviously take your reading very seriously. Tell me, do you do any writing yourself?'

'I used to write a good deal,' said the thin young man, 'when I was in better health. But it was a struggle. Most of it was only good for the fire. More recently, I've had to write stories to pay the doctor's bills.'

'Perhaps you would like to read some of my stories,' he said, seeing that I was interested. And he produced a couple of pages of small black, wiggly handwriting. 'You know German?' he asked hopefully.

'Not really,' I said. 'Well, a few words perhaps.' And I tried in vain to decipher it. Then I became aware that someone was shaking me (ripple dissolve). The young man has gone and Dorothy is trying to tell me something.

Wake up! There are some customers here. You were going to talk to them about short stories and essays.

Right! Sorry about that. Yes, short stories and essays. What's the difference? Well, the obvious answer is that although they are both short pieces of prose, one is fiction and the other is fact. But look more closely and you may agree with me that there is a good deal of overlap. A short story can be a way of expressing an argument or a point of view, and an essayist often tells stories from personal experience. Either way, you can learn a lot about the author's personality from a few pages. Two of my favourite writers of short pieces are Franz Kafka and George Orwell. Both are regarded as having identified, and in Kafka's case prophesied, some of the worst aspects of the twentieth century. Both have had their names turned into adjectives which you will find in the dictionary – Orwellian and Kafkaesque. These words are used in a political sense to describe a world ruled by oppression and fear where everyone is under suspicion and individual freedom is denied. And yet the more you read them, the more you discover that both Orwell and Kafka are telling you as much about their inner lives as about the outer world of politics and society.

THE COMPLETE SHORT STORIES by Franz Kafka (1905–1924)

Let's start with Kafka. He was born in Prague in 1883, and died of tuberculosis in 1924, aged 40. He belonged to·the Jewish community and he wrote in German. He left three unfinished novels, of which the best known is *The Trial* (*see* Chapter 5). However, he also wrote many fascinating short stories throughout his life. These days, Kafka would have been regarded as a suitable case for psychotherapy (probably CBT). He had overwhelming feelings of being totally inadequate both mentally and physically. He had a very self-confident and bullying father who is generally held responsible for making him feel inferior and guilty. However, this is probably not the whole story, human development being more complicated than that. Many of his stories are told from the point of view of an animal whom he uses to embody his own feelings about himself and his relationships. The best-known animal story is *The Metamorphosis*, in which a young salesman wakes up one morning to find that he has turned into a giant insect. His family regard their transformed son with dismay and disgust. Although his sister is kind to him for a while, they all end up conspiring to get rid of him. The story can be interpreted on all sorts of levels (one of the great joys of reading Kafka), but it is clear that he is also telling us that he feels no better than an insect himself. Other animal personas include a dog, an ape, a mole and a mouse.

The dog tries to be a scientist, investigating where food comes from, but ends up becoming overwhelmed by a kind of religious experience (God is often to be found haunting Kafka's writing, and is usually teasingly inaccessible). The ape gives 'A report to an academy' of how he learned to impersonate human beings (the key to this was drinking alcohol). The mole constructs a complicated labyrinthine burrow in which to hide from an enemy who is nevertheless tunnelling relentlessly towards him. And then there is Josephine, the singing mouse, a wonderful portrait of a prima donna, written when Kafka was dying. Although the protagonists are animals, there is no Disney-style sentimentality in these stories. They are all metaphors of the human predicament, and they all show us just how it felt to be Franz Kafka. I must add that although the stories sound rather grim, they are also very funny. Kafka used to laugh out loud while reading them to friends, and I sometimes do the same. You will find all of these and many other weird and wonderful tales in *Franz Kafka: the Complete Stories*. Missing is Kafka's *Letter to his Father* (written in 1919 but never delivered). This is a very revealing and moving document, but is it a short story? Look for it on the internet (www.Kafka-Franz/KAFKA-letter.htm).

ESSAYS by George Orwell (1931–1946)

Now let us consider George Orwell. He is most famous for his two late novels, *1984* and *Animal Farm*, but he also wrote some classic essays, of which a very good selection has been published by Penguin. Orwell has been one of my heroes ever since I first read him in my teens. He has a very plain, direct style which immediately grabs your attention and makes you feel that a good friend is telling you something very interesting and important. Born Eric Blair (no relation) in 1903, he was sent to Eton, although his parents could barely afford it, being posh but poor. He spent some years getting to know the British Empire at first hand as a member of the Imperial Police in Burma, and then fought in the Spanish Civil War. These experiences turned him into a journalist and a socialist as well as a novelist. One of the things he liked to do was to dive down into the lower depths of the class system and conduct his own sociological research. This produced books such as *Down and Out in Paris and London* and *The Road to Wigan Pier*, in which he gives vivid descriptions of living with poor and destitute people in the 1930s. The Penguin essays provide excellent examples of his writing on a variety of topics. From his period in Burma come the famous essays 'Shooting an Elephant' and 'A Hanging.' In 'The Spike' we find him dressed as a tramp spending a night with his fellow dossers in a 'common lodging house.' Despite his undercover disguise, the warden of the establishment recognises him as a 'gent', who he assumes is experiencing severe financial problems ('bloody bad luck, guv'nor'). While we are on the low-life stories, every doctor should read Orwell's account of a stay in a ghastly hospital in Paris, entitled 'How the Poor Die.' You will never complain about the hygiene of NHS hospitals again. These essays read like reports from the front line, but doubts have been raised about how much really happened to him and how much was imagined or at least embellished. Are they essays or stories? Who cares? We are being told some sort of truth that may be more important than the bare facts. Then there are Orwell's literary essays, the best of which is the one on Charles Dickens, which gets to the heart of the great man's enduring appeal and why we hold him in such affection despite his tendency to sentimentality. *And stereotyped portraits of women* (thank you, Dorothy).

Of course, there are also the essays about politics, socialism and what it means to be English. Many of these were written in the middle of World War Two. 'The Lion and the Unicorn' begins with the following arresting sentence: 'As I write, highly civilised human beings are flying overhead, trying to kill me.' Is being English the same now as it was in 1940? You'll have to read the essay and decide for yourself.

Orwell strongly believed that if the post-war world didn't produce a social revolution in Britain, we would have fought in vain. Although he was a champion of democratic socialism, he hated the totalitarian version imposed by Stalin, and also the way in which politicians manipulated language in order to conceal the truth. We owe to Orwell the concepts of Newspeak and Doublethink. You can hear just what he meant any time you listen to politicians being interviewed on the *Today* programme on BBC Radio 4.

So take a copy of Orwell's essays and browse through them, choosing any that appeal to you. And if you want some advice about how to write good honest English prose, you'll find no better guide than 'Politics and the English Language.'

CHAPTER 7

Books and the cinema

Great bookshop scenes from the movies: No. 1

From *The Big Sleep* (USA, 1946, director Howard Hawks).

Philip Marlowe, private investigator (alias Humphrey Bogart) is seen outside the door of an urban bookshop. Painted on the door are the words 'AJ Geiger, Rare Books, Deluxe Editions.' Bogart puts on a pair of shades and turns up the brim of his fedora to make himself look like a rare book collector. He is really seeking information about Geiger, the shop's sinister proprietor. As Bogart enters the shop, a little bell tinkles. The shelves are filled with leather-bound, expensive-looking rare books. Behind the counter is the unfriendly Agnes:

Agnes: Can I be of any assistance?

Bogart: Yes, would you happen to have a Ben Hur 1860?

Agnes: A what?

Bogart: I said would you happen to have a Ben Hur 1860?

Agnes: Oh, a first edition?

Bogart: No, no-no, no, no, no. The third, the third. The one with the erratum on page 116.

Agnes: I'm afraid not.

Bogart: How about a Chevalier Audubon 1840, full set, of course?

Agnes: Not at the moment.

Bogart: (looking at her over his specs) You do sell books? Hmm?

Agnes: (with Brooklyn whine, indicating shelves) Well whadda these look like – grapefruit?

This is by way of an introduction to our new **film section** which will be in this cosy little corner. Dorothy is already clearing a few shelves and putting up some posters to entice the film buffs. And we have ordered some of the British Film Institute's excellent BFI Film Classics series to start off with. Each of these attractive little books consists of a monograph on a favourite classic film by a well-known critic, either amateur or professional. Titles so far include *The Wizard of Oz* by Salman Rushdie, *The Seventh Seal* by Melvyn Bragg and, of course, *The Big Sleep* by David Thomson. Each essay offers an analysis of what the film is about, some intriguing revelations about how it was made, and a very personal appreciation from someone who has seen it many times. Each book is generously illustrated with stills from the film.

And now, with the swiftest of cuts here comes:

Great bookshop scenes from the movies: No. 2

Strangely enough, this scene also comes from *The Big Sleep* (directed by Howard Hawks, 1946) and it follows directly after Great Bookshop Scene No. 1. Humphrey Bogart is now in the Acme Book Shop across the street and it's pouring with rain. He is again talking to a young female assistant, but this one is wearing glasses and is less intimidating:

Bogart: Know anything about rare books?

Girl: You could try me?

Bogart: Would you happen to have a Ben Hur 1860, third edition with a duplicated line on page 116? Or a Chevalier Audubon 1840?

(*She licks her lips, looks thoughtful, and casually consults a large reference book on the counter*)

Girl: Nobody would. There isn't one.

Bogart: The girl in Geiger's bookshop didn't know that.

Girl: Oh – I see. You begin to interest me. Vaguely.

Bogart: I'm private dick on a case. Perhaps I'm asking too much. (*He wants a description of Geiger.*) Although it doesn't seem too much to me. Somehow.

Girl (smiling archly): Well, Geiger's in his early 40s, medium height, Charlie Chan mustache, well dressed, wears a black hat, affects a knowledge of antiques and hasn't any. Oh yes, I think his left eye is glass.

Bogart (admiringly): You would make a good cop.

Girl: Thanks. Going to wait for him to come out? We don't close for another hour. It's raining pretty hard.

Bogart: I got my car (flash of realisation). Hey, that's right, it is, isn't it? You know it just happens I got a bottle of pretty good rye in my pocket. I'd a lot rather get wet in here.

Girl (smiling collusively): Well. (*She closes the shop door and, turning to face him, pulls the blind down, with the merest suggestion of a little wiggle as she straightens up.*) Looks like we're closed for the rest of the afternoon . . .

Dorothy loves that scene. She keeps wanting us to role-play it. I tell her I'm too busy. Before we leave *The Big Sleep*, I must tell you that it was based on the novel by the brilliant, originally British thriller writer, Raymond Chandler. The script was entrusted to a powerful team, which included William Faulkner (*see* Chapter 5). Fortunately, they decided to leave in a lot of Chandler's original words, especially in the two bookshop scenes and the wonderful interview that Philip Marlowe (Humphrey Bogart) has with General Sternwood in the tropical heat of the General's conservatory. 'Do you like orchids, Mr Marlowe? Nasty things. Their flesh is like the flesh of men. Their odour has the rotten sweetness of corruption.' Ugh!

Let's move on to Paris and:

Great bookshop scenes from the movies: No. 3

Boudu Saved from Drowning (Boudu sauvé des eaux) (directed by Jean Renoir, 1932).

Jean Renoir, son of the impressionist painter Auguste Renoir, was one of the great movie directors of all time, and this modest black and white film is a masterpiece of comedy and poetry. Boudu is a shaggy and obstreperous tramp who tries to drown himself by jumping off a bridge into the river Seine. He is rescued by a kindly middle-class antiquarian bookseller who has observed the drama through his telescope. The bookseller (Monsieur Lestingois) has a lovely old shop (with house attached) in the Latin Quarter overlooking the Pont des Arts. Boudu is carried inside to be given some rather old-fashioned resuscitation (using the Holger–Neilsen method if I am not mistaken), followed by some dry clothes and a meal. He is even invited to stay on as a guest. Is he grateful? Not in the least. He is rude and uncouth and resists all attempts to introduce him to the bourgeois lifestyle. He demands sardines which he then eats with his fingers, he cleans his shoes on the best bedspread, and he seduces both Madame Lestingois and Marie Anne, the housemaid. He is of course a free spirit. Boudu is played by the legendary French character actor Michel Simon in a performance that is both entertaining and slightly scary. But he is not much of a reader. So where do the books come in? Well, the shop is full of wonderful leather-bound volumes, and the occasional customer does appear. When a poor student asks the price of a book by Voltaire and is unable to afford it, the good-natured bookseller gives it to him as a present, and adds another one for good measure.

'But you don't know me,' says the student. 'I know you,' replies Lestingois, 'your name is Youth.'

Boudu's relationship to Voltaire is more problematic. When he is scolded for trying to spit on the floor, he surreptitiously hawks between the pages of a probably priceless first edition of the great writer's *Physiologie de Mariage*. Lestingois is shaken and horrified by this despicable act. Boudu's contempt for marriage is made more apparent when he escapes from his own wedding party by falling out of the boat and swimming strongly away from the entanglements of middle-class respectability.

The film, which is beautiful to look at as well as very funny, was shown at the National Film Theatre's Renoir season a few years ago. If you missed that, a very good print is available on DVD. I can also recommend the delightful BFI monograph on the film by Richard Boston, which celebrates the joys of *Boudu* and free associates happily about its links with Greek philosophy, books, rivers, impressionism, Shakespeare and the Marx Brothers. See the film, read the book. Let Boudu enter and disrupt your inner life!

* * * * *

David Thomson is one of our best writers about American film. In 2004 he produced a book called *The Whole Equation: a History of Hollywood*, in which he tells the story of the dream factory from the early monochrome silents to the colossal blockbusters of today. He also tries to find an answer to the question 'Is cinema an art or an industry?' The phrase 'dream factory' sums up the contradiction. As Thomson points out, if you write a novel it remains your intellectual and artistic property and you can do what you like with it, including deciding whether or not it will have a happy ending. But try to turn your story into a movie and you soon find that a large number of other people want to take over the controls. There's the director and the actors, of course, not to mention the cinematographer. There have to be compromises. But the person who really decides how your movie will look and whether it will appear at all is the man with the money.

How did this happen? Before the First World War, moving pictures were just a novelty, exhibited in seedy little theatres called 'nickelodeons', because a nickel was the price of admission. Then along came Louis B Mayer and a group of other 'foreign' businessmen (mostly refugees from Europe) who were able to see into the future. They knew that people would be seduced in their millions by the magical experience of sitting in the dark and being told stories in the form of moving pictures. Soon Mayer and his colleagues were controlling the distribution of the new product, and the final step was to start making the films themselves. The business of Metro-Goldwyn-Mayer and the other studios was to churn out a picture a week and keep them flowing into the theatres all over the country where the nickels and the dollars could be collected. So was Louis B Mayer just a ruthless entrepreneur or was there a touch of the artist in his make-up, too? He loved storytelling, he certainly loved actresses, and he loved the whole process of movie-making, which he supervised very closely. But the real artists in the early days were people like DW Griffith, Charlie Chaplin and Erich von Stroheim, who were struggling with varying degrees of success to get their own imaginative visions on to the screen. Most submitted to being owned by the studio, while Stroheim ruined himself by recklessly spending the studio's money on magnificent but unrealistic projects such as *Greed*, which was originally intended to run for hours. Chaplin and some of his friends were wise enough to set up their own production company (United Artists).

Thomson traces the careers of all the legendary producers, directors and stars. He praises their (occasional) artistic achievements, but also takes care to remind us how much everything cost, how much everyone was paid and how many cinema seats were sold each week across the United States. The peak attendance was in 1946, when the average weekly attendance was 100 million. Sales went up with the coming of sound and Technicolor. Then they took a nosedive in the 1950s with the coming of television, only to revive gradually through the appeal of blockbusters such as *Star Wars* and *The Lord of the Rings*.

So what, in the end, is the cinema? Thomson's conclusion seems to be that it contains the potential for artistic creation, but because of the need to balance art against the money on the other side of the equation, art is rarely achieved. How many Hollywood films approach the artistic level of the great classic novels? Only a tiny proportion of the total output, but enough to give us a lot of pleasure every time we revisit them. I would hate to be without *The Gold Rush*, *Some Like it Hot* and *The Godfather*, to name just a few.

Cinemeducation (2005)

Hollywood movies also have a role to play in medical education. If you would like to know more, it is all explained in a book called *Cinemeducation: a Comprehensive Guide to Using Film in Medical Education*, edited by Matthew Alexander, Patricia Lenahan and Ann Pavlov.

The idea is that films frequently tell us stories of illness or emotional conflict. They show us how these crises affect our relationships with each other, and with our doctors, in a way that is easily accessible and enjoyable. Movies have an appeal that PowerPoint just can't match. Having caught your students' attention with a film extract, you can then easily involve them in a lively discussion about the issues that have been raised. Hopefully this will lead to further reflection about how patients feel, and to a general increase in empathy and emotional intelligence in a cinematically educated generation of doctors.

The approach of *Cinemeducation* is topic driven. The authors aim to list the key scenes from the most appropriate film for every subject in the psychosocial medicine curriculum. For each sequence they provide a helpful list of 'trigger questions' to get the discussion going. We start with The Life Cycle (child and adolescent development through family dynamics and sexuality to old age and death). The next section deals with mental health problems (depression, anxiety, eating disorders and schizophrenia). The last two sections cover the doctor–patient relationship and the needs of specific populations. Thus, if you wanted to teach the psychosocial aspects of diabetes care, you would opt for *Steel Magnolias*, starting with the scene in the hairdressers, 18 minutes 37 seconds from the beginning, where the ill-fated heroine has an attack of hypoglycaemia hours before her wedding. If generalised anxiety is your chosen theme, you can show your students the brain tumour scene in *Hannah and her Sisters* and then have a discussion about how best to help Woody Allen to be less neurotic (now there's a challenge).

If you want to try out the method, the book will be incredibly useful in accurately guiding you to the film sequences that you need and prompting you with questions for discussion. Personally, I have a problem with this particular approach to the use of film, and it goes back to David Thomson's questions about whether a movie is a work of art or a product. It seems to me that if we show our students films, we should introduce them to the best that the medium can offer. And I'm sorry to say that the great majority of the films used in *Cinemeducation* are artistically not the finest. They are often very sentimental, and I feel that they are aiming to manipulate the emotions of the audience rather than to communicate a personal vision. Our learners see this sort of thing on television or at their local multi-screen every day of the week. Why not show them classics like *The Seventh Seal* or *Les Enfants du Paradis* or *A Matter of Life and Death* – wonderful films they might otherwise never see? That would be different, but very educational.

Have you seen . . .? A personal introduction to 1000 films by David Thomson (2008)

This was a 1000-page birthday present from my daughter. She knows what I like, and this was a welcome treat. It is David Thomson's personal account of his 1000 best films. I say 'best' films, but he admits that among the masterpieces are some 'oddities and guilty pleasures, with just a few disasters.' So are they really the 1000 movies he most wanted to write about? Are all film viewings a kind of guilty pleasure? Let's investigate that one as I dive addictively into the book. The first thing I notice is that the films are arranged in alphabetical order with no attempt to rank them in order of merit, as is done in other Top 1000 books. I approve of Thomson's decision. How can you possibly make such arbitrary decisions on films that please or shake you up in so many different ways? All the same, there is something irresistible about the Top Ten lists, and even Thomson succumbs to talking about them in his introduction. He mentions that the *Sight and Sound* poll of critics and directors (which appears once a decade) has put *Citizen Kane* at Number 1 from 1962 to 2002. Now some of you will be saying 'What, that old thing?' or even 'Citizen *Who*?'

You may well prefer the smoother, slicker, modern movies with glorious colour and amazing special effects. You have a choice of heart-warming love stories, spectacular science fiction and/or sickening depictions of violence.

Are my prejudices showing here? Maybe they are because, with a few exceptions, I prefer the oldies, especially the ones made between 1930 and 1960. David Thomson admits that his 1000 films include a very high proportion of those, too, and wonders if it's because the movies you see when you are young have the most lasting effect on the heart. He and I are about the same age, so if that is true, it's no wonder our tastes tend to coincide. Many of the films that I love best I first saw as a student. Yet, curiously, some of the ones I only discovered in the last 20 years belong to the decade before I was born. I suspect that there is something about seeing people on the screen who remind you of your parents when they were young. Although I will maintain that even without the roseate glow of nostalgia and the inescapable logic of dollar-book Freud, the classic oldies really are better than anything that has come out since. After all, they have endured.

Thomson writes very well about his movies. I read greedily through all my favourites to start with, without putting the book down. I shall return to the ones I remember less well or have never seen. I note with pleasure that even when he has written about a film elsewhere, he finds a different take or a different telling phrase this time round. And some of his opinions have mellowed since he wrote his *Biographical Dictionary of Film*. He is much more appreciative of Ingmar Bergman, which I note with approval. The other directors we both love and revere include Jean Renoir, Howard Hawks, Billy Wilder and Alfred Hitchcock. My top ten (you will not be surprised to see their names appearing again) would have to include *Wild Strawberries, La Grande Illusion, Bringing up Baby, Vertigo* and, of course, *Citizen Kane*. And if you haven't already fallen under its spell, try, before you die, to see Renoir's 40-minute *Partie de Campagne*, the ultimate story of a pretty girl on a swing and a love that might have been.

CHAPTER 8

Biography and memoirs

We will start with two biography reviews kindly contributed by Mary Salinsky.

SAMUEL PEPYS: THE UNEQUALLED SELF by Claire Tomalin (2003)

Any biography of Pepys has to deal with two related difficulties – avoiding merely rehearsing the Diary, and writing about those parts of his life that are not covered by the Diary, so that a picture of the whole man and the whole life emerges. In *Samuel Pepys: the Unequalled Self*, Claire Tomalin has most ably succeeded.

Tomalin devotes 13 of the biography's 26 chapters to the period covered by the Diary. For information on the earlier and later parts of Pepys' life, she uses many contemporary and modern sources that provide some picture of the rest of his life, but they are thin pickings compared with the intimate and vivid material in the Diary. Sometimes she is able to use the Diary to throw light on earlier events, such as Pepys recalling that he had been 'a great Roundhead when I was a boy.' She employs other contemporary sources for her account of his operation for the removal of a large kidney stone, but finds in the Diary that he sought information and anatomical explanations from the doctors who attended him. This 'cutting for the stone' probably saved his life, and when he eventually recovered it gave him years free from the pain. The pain recurred towards the end of his life, and Tomalin tells how the post-mortem found a mass of further stones in his left kidney. She shows how the need for patronage in seventeenth-century life forced Pepys to accommodate himself to it as his employers negotiated their way from Republican officials to Royal servants, taking Pepys along with them. He always knew that his professional success was due as much to favour from kings of whom he was deeply critical, as to his own abilities.

Tomalin organises the material of the Diary according to themes, but also keeps the story moving along chronologically. She selects small touches from the Diary to light up the person and the times. For example, during the Great Fire, Pepys wrote a letter to his father but could not post it because the post office had burned down. When the Diary ends, because Pepys feared he was going blind, Tomalin stresses not only the loss for us as readers, but also the loss for Pepys himself as he ended it. These losses are all the more poignant because, as Tomalin explains, Pepys was not in fact going blind, and his eyesight deteriorated no further.

We are given a lively account of the physical appearance of the Diary, with its careful ink shorthand and occasional words in longhand, including bowdlerised Spanish and French words for the naughty bits. We also learn how the Diary was eventually laboriously deciphered, while all the time the key to the shorthand that Pepys had used sat in the primer on the same library shelves.

Claire Tomalin writes beautifully, and this book is a delight to read. It will send me back to the Diary with renewed keenness.

JANE AUSTEN by Carol Shields (2001)

Carol Shields tells us in her bibliographical note that she became curious about Jane Austen's life as soon as she began to read her novels. This is her own way of satisfying that curiosity. She sets about it as one novelist writing the biography of another. She wants principally to show how the novels came to be written. She traces Jane Austen's education – boarding school without much intellectual content, and the run of her father's library – and discusses the novel-reading habits of the Austen family. She describes how the new literary form of the novel had recently become popular and was enjoyed, probably uncritically, by all the Austen family. She describes the young Jane's early ideas about becoming a novelist and her first efforts at writing, which were tried out on her family and encouraged by her father. She also considers the emotional atmosphere in which Jane Austen grew up, and her growing realisation that she was completely dependent on others – chiefly her male relatives – for the economic and social necessities of life. She could marry, become a governess, or stay at home with her mother. Carol Shields argues that this reality for all women at this time, together with Jane Austen's experiences of being sent away from home in childhood, account for the notion of home as a refuge and a place of love and acceptance that she finds to be the principal theme in Jane Austen's novels.

Carol Shields explains the long gap in Jane Austen's writing between 1800 and 1810 by the emotional, economic and practical difficulties that she experienced when the family moved to Bath. Her father's death led to poverty for the family, and many changes of lodging. It was only on being re-established in a village in a familiar part of the country that Jane Austen was able to draw on 'the delight of my life', the social interactions of a few village families, to enable her to continue writing.

Carol Shields comments illuminatingly on the difficulties of writing in general – for instance, the need for a balance between solitude and social contact – and shows how these affected Jane Austen, who was never alone and whose work was refined by the comments of a close and familiar group of people. She refers to the need for the author to believe in the worth of what she writes, reflecting on how Jane Austen was able, because of her belief, to write *Emma* immediately after *Mansfield Park* had met with little appreciation.

Through this biography, I now feel that I 'know' Jane Austen better than I did, as Carol Shields has made her subject so vivid. She has illuminatingly explored the way that Jane Austen's life and circumstances were reflected in the novels. However, as Carol Shields comments:

> What is known of Jane Austen's life will never be enough to account for the greatness of her novels . . . The two 'accounts' – the life and the work – will always lack congruency and will sometimes appear to be in complete contradiction.

Carol Shields has, however, brought the two most revealingly together, encouraging me to go back to the six novels.

Thank you, Mary.

* * * * * *

1599: A YEAR IN THE LIFE OF WILLIAM SHAKESPEARE
by James Shapiro (2005)

Now I'd like to recommend this thoroughly enjoyable and informative little book that covers a single year in the life of Shakespeare. It's an easy year to remember, being the one before the turn of the century, and it was an important one for William.

In his PDP, if he had kept one, he would have been able to note the successful completion and performance of *Henry the Fifth*, *Julius Caesar* and *As You Like It*. And the first draft of *Hamlet* written. Not a bad year's work considering that his company, the Chamberlain's Men, had also had to pull down their theatre in North London, transport it across London and re-erect it (as The Globe) on the South Bank.

The author of *1599*, James Shapiro, is a professor of literature at Columbia University, so he is well able to throw some light on the plays and their inner meanings. He also gives us a very immediate sense of what it would have been like to live and work in the Elizabethan theatre. The other thing he does is to set the writing and performing of the plays in their social and political context. Can you remember what happened in history in 1599? The Earl of Essex had taken an army over to Ireland to subdue the rebels. The troops were urged on with a certain amount of patriotic fervour (think *Henry the Fifth*). Elizabeth was getting old and there was anxiety about who would succeed her. Philip of Spain was rumoured to be sending another Armada and being abetted by English conspirators (*Julius Caesar?*).

I was also intrigued by the way the plays were shaped by the resources that William had at his disposal. At the beginning of 1599, his chief clown, Will Kemp, decided to leave the company and so Falstaff, who was his creation, does not appear in *Henry the Fifth* (although he is mentioned). And what about those boy actors who took the women's parts? The plays often have two featured female characters (for example, Portia and Calpurnia in *Julius Caesar*, Rosalind and Celia in *As You Like it*, Gertrude and Ophelia in *Hamlet*), probably because there were just two excellent boys in the company. They must have been very talented, but we don't know their names. And the first Rosalind must have been a real star. There are many more revelations and speculations about Shakespeare's life and work in this book, and I finished it with a feeling of satisfaction – as if I had just spent a year with the Chamberlain's Men and their resident genius.

A SHAPE OF MY OWN by Grace Bowman (2006)

How do you cope with patients who have anorexia nervosa? I expect that, like me, you find them desperately worrying and very hard to engage with. We have read all the theories and the guidelines, but how can we know what it feels like to be a teenager trapped by her own determination in a thin, shrinking body? Well, here is a book that might help us. It's called *A Shape of My Own* and it's by Grace Bowman, who developed the eating disorder when she was 18. Her first sentence is 'If I share a secret with you, do you promise to tell everyone?' Well, yes, of course, so what is the secret? It's more like a secret inner world which the reader is invited to enter and explore. To begin with, Grace relates her story in the third person, as if she herself is now someone else (which to some extent she is). Grace has a normal, happy childhood. She moves from child to teenager to . . . anorexic. At school she wants to be top, she wants to be popular and she wants to be in control. At the age of 18 she develops glandular fever and is off school for six weeks. She starts to worry about her A levels. She passes her driving test but is terrified when she tries to drive on her own. Reasserting control, she formulates her personal development plan: Got to do well. Got to get top marks. Got to be pretty. Got to be popular . . . *Got to be thin.*

We watch in fascination and dismay as Grace eats less and exercises more. She knows the number of calories in every spoonful of low-fat Pot Noodle. Her weight drops from eight stone to seven and to six and below. The secret plan is working. Apart from being cold all the time she feels fine. But people are beginning to notice, and soon she is dragged off to the doctor. At this point the authorial voice interrupts and gives us some theoretical background on what is currently known or believed about anorexia. After that Grace is able to tell at least some of the story in the first person, in her own voice. She tells us how it felt to be 'young, thin and aloof.' She takes care to point out that she can't speak for everyone – this is only the way anorexia was for her. But her report from the field is a kind of ethnography and, as we have seen, a single case study can be more illuminating than a lot of facts and figures.

Like most anorexics, Grace resists the attempts of family and friends to put food on her plate. She is bored or irritated by the intrusions of 'the white-coats.' So how does she escape from her anorexic prison in the end? She simply decides one day to change her secret plan. To avoid going into hospital she will gradually eat a little more and accept the offer of a place to do English at Cambridge. Of course there are ups and downs, but that is how the turning point was achieved. I still don't understand why people have anorexia but, having been let into Grace's secret world, I think I have a much better idea how it feels – cold, detached, secret, proud, and afraid.

ACCORDING TO QUEENEY by **Beryl Bainbridge (2001)**

From now on the distinction between biography and fiction starts to blur as our life chroniclers imagine their way into their subjects' lives to give us a more vivid portrait. I think this biographical novel must have been one of the best books published in 2001, even though the Booker Prize judges chose to ignore it (they didn't even put it in the final six). It tells the story of the complicated relationship between Samuel Johnson and the Thrale family over a period of 20 years (1765–1784). Johnson, you will remember, was the famous writer and lexicographer whose witticisms and crushing put-downs were faithfully recorded by James Boswell. Another very important person in his life was Mrs Hester Thrale, the wife of a wealthy London brewer. Johnson had a considerable crush on this attractive, vivacious woman (possibly they even had an affair), and in his later years he was practically adopted by the whole family. 'Queeney' is the nickname of the Thrales' eldest daughter, for whom the old boy also had a soft spot. He first encounters her as a one-year-old when 'coming face to face with his boots on the bend of the stairs she had neither screamed nor scrambled past, simply stared gravely up at him.' Johnson says 'Sweeting', and Queeney says 'Da-da', before crawling on her way. After that, says Beryl Bainbridge, 'he was inclined to believe he was part of a family.'

Compared with Boswell's biography, this book gives us a picture of the great scholar as a much more human person – vulnerable, lonely and frequently touching. It's true he still roars aggressively at people and makes scathing rejoinders, but afterwards he is very worried that he has hurt the victim's feelings. Often he is not a very comfortable person to be with. He is large and ponderous, his shirt is hanging out, his wig doesn't fit, and he is constantly making hooting noises and twitching his legs (Tourette syndrome?). He also suffers from fearful bouts of depression, described in Churchillian terms as a 'Black Dog' which sometimes leaps on his chest. However, when not depressed he can be great fun at a party. Samuel is pathetically dependent on Mrs Thrale, and becomes very upset when she appears to be indifferent to him. While I was enjoying all these revelations about Johnson and the Thrales I kept wondering how much of it was true and how much Beryl had made up. It was impossible to tell, and in the end I decided that I didn't care. Although the title suggests that everything is seen from Queeney's point of view, this is not consistently the case – perhaps the book should be called 'According to Beryl.' But I'm sure you will like Queeney, who grows up to be a bright observant girl who is clearly very fond of her mother's eccentric and brilliant companion.

ARTHUR AND GEORGE by Julian Barnes (2005)

Have you ever had occasion to notice that your life has become strangely intertwined with someone else's? This happens to Arthur and George, the eponymous heroes of Julian Barnes' latest biographical novel. Arthur is Sir Arthur Conan Doyle, the famous late Victorian author and creator of

Sherlock Holmes. George is a young Staffordshire solicitor who is wrongfully convicted and imprisoned for a series of irrational attacks on horses. Arthur reads about poor George's plight, realises at once that he must be innocent, and deploys all the skills of his own fictional detective to get him released and vindicated. These events actually happened. We are assured that all quotations from letters and newspapers are genuine. Of course one can't be sure that the descriptions of Arthur and George's inner lives are authentic, but the writing is so good that I was completely convinced. We begin with parallel accounts of the boyhood and family life of the two men. Arthur's father is an alcoholic but his mother is a tower of strength, and he has all the advantages of a Scottish middle-class upbringing. George's father is a vicar, and we gradually discover that he is from India. At school he is teased and told that he is 'not a right sort' because of his colour and his strange surname (Edalji), which everyone almost deliberately mispronounces.

George is quiet but determined. He goes to college and qualifies as a solicitor. He writes a book, *Railway Law*, 'for the man in the train.' Meanwhile, in far away Edinburgh, Arthur studies medicine and has a brief unsuccessful career as an ophthalmologist before Sherlock Holmes takes over his life. Back in Staffordshire, George's father receives a series of weird anonymous letters. In the surrounding countryside someone is creeping up on horses and slashing their bellies with a knife. The wounds are superficial, but sometimes the poor animals bleed to death. The attacks seem pointless, and George seems like the last person in the county to do such a thing. But the letters hint that he is the perpetrator, and the police seem horribly eager to bang him up. Is this racism or just perverse stupidity? We feel deeply for George as we experience with him his trial, conviction and sojourn in prison, where he conducts himself with dignity, despite his inner anguish. It is so desperately unfair. Then Sir Arthur rides to the rescue, determined to 'make a noise.' He meets George, noses around the scene of the crime, and has an exciting confrontational interview with the Chief Constable, who has been George's chief persecutor. Evidence is uncovered and will be laid before you. George is released and pardoned, but the verdict of the jury cannot be reversed. Sir Arthur's activities made the Edalji case seem like an English Dreyfus affair, and led to the foundation of the Court of Criminal Appeal. The latter part of the book is less gripping, but it has a gentle appeal. Arthur's invalid wife dies, and he finally marries his secret sweetheart, Jean, with whom he has had a passionate but completely chaste relationship for ten years. He becomes increasingly interested in spiritualism. George is sceptical but respectful of his hero's beliefs. He is invited to Sir Arthur's wedding, and the two continue to meet occasionally, but they remain in different worlds and never become close friends. *Arthur and George* is an unusual book, always interesting, sometimes exciting and often moving. I think you will enjoy it.

IN COLD BLOOD: A TRUE ACCOUNT OF MULTIPLE MURDER AND ITS CONSEQUENCES by Truman Capote (1966)

If you saw the excellent film *Capote*, you might like to read this book that Truman Capote wrote about the two young men who brutally murdered a Kansas family in 1959. The book was called *In Cold Blood*, and when it was published in 1962 it caused quite a sensation, partly because of its lurid subject matter but mainly because readers were unsettled by its mixture of truth and fiction. Previously, it seems, writers did not embellish reports of true events with invented details of what the villains might have said to each other and what the detective had for breakfast. Capote changed all that, and such books no longer surprise us. However, he is an exceptionally good writer, and his book is a compelling blend of reportage and imagined dialogue. We start with a description of the unfortunate Clutter family, mother and father and two adolescent children, leading innocent untroubled lives in a prosperous Kansas home. We are then introduced to the two killers, Richard Hickock and Perry Smith, as their car heads ominously across Kansas towards their date with the victims. Why did they kill four perfectly nice people whom they had never met, all for a haul of 'between 40 and 50 dollars'? As the story unfolds, we get to know them very well, and it's so well written that we cease to bother about how much of their conversation is based on fact. According to the film, Capote became very involved with the killers while they were on Death Row, and helped to find lawyers for their appeals. But he also needed them to be executed so that his book could have a neat conclusion. He was even allowed to witness (and hence describe) the hangings. Talk about cold blood! None of this authorial influence on events is evident in the book, which presents itself as an objective account, or in the author's words, 'a narrative form that employed all the techniques of fiction but was, nevertheless, immaculately factual.'

UNTOLD STORIES by Alan Bennett (2005)

Lastly comes an autobiographical treat, as tasty and filling as a good fruitcake. It's a thick, rich, 600-page slab of Alan Bennett's assorted writings which he has called *Untold Stories*. Perfect for a long train journey or a night when you can't sleep and need some comfort reading. Now I'm going to confide in you. I have always felt a strong affinity with Mr Bennett. We both grew up in Leeds in the 1940s, although he had a six-year start on me. We both took the entrance exam for the Grammar School (I passed but he failed and had to go to Leeds Modern, which was also a grammar school but not so posh). My dad died of a heart attack in 1974 (so did his), and both our mothers suffered from depression. We both went to Oxford. He sprang to fame in *Beyond the Fringe*, wrote some brilliant plays, declined a knighthood and became a national treasure. Meanwhile I became a humble little country doctor. The rest is history. We have never actually met, but I feel I know Alan like an old friend because the Leeds he talks about in his memoirs is my Leeds – a drab, smoke-blackened provincial city enlivened for us both by the renaissance splendour of the County Arcade and the Yorkshire Symphony Orchestra playing Brahms and Beethoven in the Town Hall. Now if you had the misfortune to be born somewhere else, don't worry. There is still plenty in this book to entertain you and to make you think 'By 'eck, that's true, our Alan, you've put your finger on it there, lad.' We start with an extended memoir of Bennett's parents and grandparents and eccentric aunties. His father was an atypical butcher – thin and introverted, and not a good mixer. As he says to his son, 'We're neither of us much in the mixing line. We were when we were first married, but you lose the knack.' Alan's dad also disliked a lot of 'splother', which was his word for the pomp and ceremony that goes with weddings and suchlike. There is a very moving and sympathetic account of his mother's recurrent depression which merged into dementia as she became older. 'Written on the Body' tells us about school days, national service and coming to terms with his sexuality. There is a good long chunk of diary (1996–2004), as well as an account of a recent brush with mortality when he developed a cancer of the colon and happily survived. Doctors on the whole get a good write-up, especially his GP in Camden (well done, Roy). And there's a lot more, including his thoughts about art treasures in the National Gallery where he was made a trustee 'to represent the man in the street.' It may seem rather a ragbag collection, but it's always absorbing because Bennett writes so well. He is brilliantly observant, and he has a special gift for capturing the tragical–comical quality of human life in perfect phrases. I know it's a heavy book, but you can have five pounds off, and isn't that a lovely picture of him on the cover in his green scarf? His Mam would have been proud.

CHAPTER 9

Non-fiction

***A SHORT HISTORY OF NEARLY EVERYTHING* by Bill Bryson (2003)**

Some of you, I know, get a bit restless with all the fiction and escapism on our shelves, and would like to read something serious and scientific. So let me introduce Bill Bryson, who has just the book for you – solidly scientific and definitely stranger than fiction. Bill made his name with travel books such as *Notes from a Small Island*. Now, after taking three years to find out all about science, he has come up with *A Short History of Nearly Everything*. This is a wonderfully entertaining and informative gallop through physics, chemistry and biology, taking in the origin and nature of the universe, elements and particles, proteins and chromosomes, the rise of life and the origin of man. I am happy to say that there is hardly any maths.

Now we doctors with our scientific education are supposed to know all this stuff, but I don't mind admitting I had forgotten most of it and failed to understand the rest. How did Bill, a complete amateur who didn't know a protein from a proton, manage to learn all this science and then put it across in such an engaging and absorbing way? The notes at the back reveal that most of his sources are other popular science writers, but he does also describe some conversations he has had with eminent professors whom he tracked down to their laboratories and museums. Along the way, there are some very enjoyable accounts of the lives of the more eccentric scientific pioneers, such as Newton, Hooke and Darwin. Another thing that makes the book enjoyable is the constant presence of the author, sharing his own fascination with the mystery of it all. He congratulates us all on being here to read the book, and points out how utterly improbable it is that human beings ever managed to emerge and evolve. As he points out, we are nothing but a mass of atoms who are not really interested in us at all. I said there wasn't any maths, but there are some awe-inspiring numbers – the vastness and emptiness of space, and the tiny dimensions of atoms which at the same time manage to be so full of nothing that other particles pass right through them. Bill finishes by reminding us that as a species we are not the people you would choose to take good care of the planet: 'It's an unnerving thought that we may be the living universe's supreme achievement and its worse nightmare simultaneously.' Bill's book is a chunky 500 pages, but it's a delight to read and you must take a copy.

HARD WORK: LIFE IN LOW-PAID BRITAIN by Polly Toynbee (2003)

Have you ever wondered whether you could survive on the national minimum wage? Be honest, do you even know how low it is? I didn't until I read this little book by Polly Toynbee, a *Guardian* journalist who specialises in social affairs. Polly has a keen intelligence and a liberal conscience that burns with a clear bright flame. In 2002, she decided to spend the six weeks of Lent supporting herself on jobs that paid around the minimum wage, which by the way was then £4.10 an hour or about £10 000 a year. To begin with, this involved moving out of her comfortable middle-class house and into a flat in a concrete block on a council estate in Clapham. Then, before she had even found a job, she had to furnish the flat and feed herself on a Jobseeker's Allowance of £53 a week. This was impossible, so she had to beg for a loan from the Social Fund to buy herself a bed, table, chairs and a cooker. We hear reports of this kind of hardship from our patients, but somehow it makes a much bigger impact if the sufferer is a fellow member of the middle class.

Polly's first job was as a hospital porter, employed by a private company, which had the contract for all non-clinical work in the hospital – that's the way it is in the NHS nowadays. The work was hard and badly organised, and mainly involved moving patients about the hospital with minimal cooperation between porters and nurses. However, the people were friendly and she was soon accepted. At the end of a 40-hour week she took home £150.67, which was not enough to pay the rent and the bills. After that came jobs as a dinner lady, an assistant in a posh nursery run by the Foreign Office, a cold calling telephone salesperson, an office cleaner, a cake packer and a care assistant in an old people's home. All of the jobs are graphically described and they make fascinating reading. In the course of six weeks Polly came across many people who were astonishingly gifted. They took pride in doing a difficult and unpleasant job well, and they were able to inspire a team spirit in other people and to make sure that essential services continued to function. At the same time they were working really hard to earn about a tenth of the income of a top journalist or a doctor. Perhaps unsurprisingly, the great majority of the low-paid workers were women. And the jobs they did were 'caring, cleaning, cooking, teaching and nursing. Things your mother did for you freely out of love.' It seems that we now expect women to be society's mothers for £4.10 an hour (£5.80 at the time of writing). Polly Toynbee has now returned to the comforts of middle-class life. But her book is an absorbing, mind-opening read and a great social document.

EMPIRE: HOW BRITAIN MADE THE MODERN WORLD
by Niall Ferguson (2003)

Now let us consider the British Empire. Was it a good thing or a bad thing? Discuss. But before you do that, let me recommend a suitable text. It's by Niall Ferguson, a respected historian who makes his subject very readable. He is also suspected of being a little too generous to the old Imperialists – but that we must judge for ourselves. The other question raised by Professor Ferguson is 'Why Britain?' How did 'an archipelago of rainy islands off the north-west coast of Europe' come to rule three-quarters of the world? The story starts in Elizabethan times when we distinguished ourselves as pirates, robbing the Spanish colonists of their South American gold by seizing their ships and raiding their ports. Next came the British 'sweet tooth.' Hungry for sugar and spices to sweeten our disgusting food and for recreational drugs to soothe us (tea, coffee and tobacco), we started setting up plantations in other people's countries. Of course we needed workers to pick the crops (which soon included cotton), and they were supplied by the slave trade.

So far the Empire appears as cruel, greedy, rapacious and merciless. But on the other side of the world, the East India Company was encouraging Indian production of cloth and providing markets for it. The trouble was that India became too important to leave to the Indians, and it became necessary to rule and govern most of it, too. Another important ingredient was the British desire to spread Christianity. Large numbers of missionaries went to Africa and India in the hope of converting the heathens and saving their souls. It was dangerous work, and many of the missionaries ended up dying of disease or being murdered by the ungrateful recipients of the gospel. However, they did succeed in providing educational opportunities and medical services, which were of lasting value. Niall Ferguson has great respect for the colonial civil servants, especially those in India. They brought to the huge areas that they administered the ideas of liberty, justice and the rule of law. They also taught their colonial subjects to speak English and to play cricket. They persuaded them to fight in our wars, but drew the line at treating them as equals, with the exception of the Australians and the Canadians, who were all white settlers. Towards the end of the nineteenth century it all got rather nasty, especially in the 'scramble' for Africa, which was carved up between the European powers. If the Africans resisted, they were easily defeated with the aid of the Maxim gun, an early machine gun that could fire 500 rounds a minute. Was the Empire a source of huge profits to the mother country? Only for a few, according to Professor Ferguson. Most people just felt pleased and proud that Britain was so powerful and important. So why did the Empire collapse? It was probably because, after two world wars, we could no longer afford it. What would the world be like if there had never been a British Empire? I shall leave you to think about that one for yourselves. *Empire* is a racy, enjoyable read, as good as a novel. There are vivid portraits of the principal characters, such as Rhodes and Livingstone. I learned a lot of history and something about why the world is still in such a sad state.

A HISTORY OF MODERN BRITAIN by Andrew Marr (2007)

How much difference does it make if we are governed by one political party or another? Was Blair better than Brown or would we get on better with Cameron? Which is more important, politics or shopping? These thoughts came to mind as I finished a large but very readable book called *A History of Modern Britain*, by the perky, likeable, former BBC political editor Andrew Marr. Andrew starts in 1945 and traces the political and social life of the country from 1945 to the very brink of current events. Did all those legendary prime ministers really make a difference? Attlee, struggling against dire national poverty to give us socialism and the welfare state, Eden collapsing under the weight of the Suez debacle, suave Harold Macmillan (who we now know was a tortured soul), technocratic people's prime minister Harold Wilson with his bad teeth and Yorkshire vowels, and of course Margaret Thatcher, perhaps the only really influential leader since Churchill.

Most of you reading this will probably not remember any prime minister before Thatcher. But I am older and I knew them all. Well, not personally, but I remember them being on the radio and in the papers. My first political memory is of my father, a staunch Labour supporter, teaching me a song called 'Vote, vote, vote for Mr Attlee.' That must have been in 1950 or 1951.

So for me, reading this book is like reading about my own life and times. And yet, although I was interested in politics, and always rooted for Labour (until I was disillusioned by Blair), my private life seemed to carry on much the same whoever was in power. Andrew Marr's book reminds me of all the great political events and the momentous decisions that governments had to make. Should we go to war over the Suez Canal? Must we devalue the pound? What about joining the Common Market? What about immigration? Did we need to keep the Falklands? The fascinating thing is that with hindsight, most of the decisions were made on the basis of grossly misleading information and a tendency, in the language of CBT, to catastrophise. To give just two examples, we didn't need the Suez Canal because large tankers could go round the Cape, and Callaghan's 1979 loan from the IMF was never needed, because the public finances were actually much better than the Treasury forecasts. On the other hand, huge changes occur simply because the people won't have it any other way. So we would probably have had the NHS even with a Conservative government in 1945. In the 1950s we just had to have cars, motorways and supermarkets. In the 1960s we needed the Beatles and clothes from Biba. Since then we have always wanted money in our pockets and bright places to spend it. But politics may be returning, warns Andrew Marr at the end. We have to do something about climate change or the party may be over. (Bank failures and economic downturn were not even a cloud on the horizon at that stage.) Meanwhile, he concludes, 'to be born British remains a wonderful stroke of luck.'

CHAPTER 10

Classic books about general practice

General practice in the UK has produced a small number of books that capture its essence and deserve to be called classics. These are the books that you earnestly recommend to your GP trainees or students ('Wonderful book, a classic, you *have* to read it'). The classic in question may even be sitting in some neglected corner of the practice library. But will our pupils actually take it down, dust it off and read it? To be honest, have we really, truly read it ourselves? Or is it, in the words of Italian novelist Italo Calvino, one of those 'books that everybody else has read, so it's as if you had read them, too.'

This is a shame, because the classics are so much more enlightening (and entertaining) than the majority of modern books about our specialty. The classic books may not be up to date, but they tell us about our history and they proclaim our core values, which we must hope will survive the nefarious plans of the politicians and healthcare experts to destroy the NHS we know and love, but don't get me started on that just now. Because I am pleased to tell you that the Green Bookshop has rescued some of these GP classic books from their dusty fate and given them a special shelf to themselves. We shall now take some of them down and give you a preview which we hope will encourage you to find and enjoy them for yourselves.

THE CITADEL by AJ Cronin (1937)

I shall present them in chronological order, starting with *The Citadel*. Yes, it's a novel and not a textbook, but as we know, some of the profoundest truths are only found in fiction. The author, AJ Cronin, was himself a doctor, and he can tell us everything we need to know about general practice in the 1920s.

A different world, you may think, but be prepared for a few surprises. Some things about general practice never seem to change.

The Citadel was a best-seller when it was first published in 1937, and it has retained a treasured place in the tribal memory of general practice. I first read it as a student, and I am still fond of it because it gives a really good, genuine account of what it's like to be a GP which hasn't dated despite all the scientific advances and the advent of the NHS. At the same time I have to admit that it's not a 'literary' novel, and the writing is often flat and conventional – although it can sometimes sweep you away on a tide of emotion.

We start with young, newly qualified Dr Andrew Manson, travelling by train to his first appointment as an assistant to an old GP in the tiny Welsh mining village of Drineffy. The year is 1924 and the NHS is only a distant dream. Manson soon finds that Dr Page, who is employing him for £20 a year (that's right, a *year*), has had a severe stroke and will never use a stethoscope again. Undeterred by the lack of a trainer, Andrew sets to work with all the enthusiasm of youth and all the evidence-based medicine he was taught at medical school. He comes across a patient with a mysterious fever, and is warned by his friend the cynical Dr Denny to 'look out for enteric in Glydar Place.' Sure enough, there is an outbreak of paratyphoid and, failing to get any response from the local public health department, the two young doctors decide to blow up the ancient town sewer, which is the cause of the trouble. Flushed (as it were) by this triumph, young Dr Manson then diagnoses a case of myxoedema madness. I remember doing the same thing myself in my first month as a GP, although I did not have to telephone to Cardiff for thyroid extract. Andrew is devoted to his working-class patients so long as they have proper illnesses. I'm afraid he has little interest in the patient's narrative and no patience at all with those who just want another bottle of the mixture. This boy wants to practise real medicine. After a while he moves to a larger town where he continues to distinguish himself. He saves a trapped miner by going down the pit and amputating his arm. He marries Christine, the loyal schoolteacher from Drineffy, who adores him and puts up with his tendency to be stroppy and difficult. He is contemptuous of the men who present themselves at his surgery demanding 'certificates' for spurious complaints (I told you the book hasn't dated), and gets himself into trouble with the committee. He does research on dust particles in the lung and is accused of cruelty to guinea pigs.

And so, fed up with small town pettiness, Andrew and Christine move to London, where everything changes. Andrew has always had a chip on his shoulder about being poor, and we see him gradually being seduced by the rich patients who delight in his straightforward manner (and his youthful good looks). He is also, I don't need to tell you, a bloody good doctor. Cronin paints a pretty scary picture of the scandalous behaviour of society doctors in 1930s London. We watch in dismay and fascination as our boy gets sucked deeper into the abyss. Then an operation that is spectacularly messed up by an incompetent surgeon brings him to his senses. He determines to throw up the high life and start a little polyclinic with two of his old mates. Thing seem to be about to get better, but there will be a tragedy and a GMC fitness-to-practise hearing before the end. Yes, *The Citadel* is a great read, even if it's not great literature. I urge you to take a copy and see for yourselves. And, by the way, there's a lovely black and white film of it, starring Robert Donat (of *The 39 Steps*) as Dr Manson and the American superstar Rosalind Russell (she was Hildy Johnson in *His Girl Friday*) as Christine. And don't miss the young Ralph Richardson as Dr Denny, the romantic surgeon and destroyer of sewers.

THE DOCTOR, HIS PATIENT AND THE ILLNESS by Michael Balint (1957)

Yes, we have all heard of this one. It's the book that launched a thousand Balint groups and taught us to ask patients about their sex lives. But what did Michael Balint really have to say in 1957 and is it still of interest today? Having recently finished re-reading it, I can report that although I have been marinated in Balint for 30 years, I found it fresh and full of surprises. The first thing that struck me was that Balint was describing a qualitative research project in which he was observing and reacting to general practice. He had a powerful conviction that some important stuff was going on between GPs and their patients (nowadays we call it the doctor–patient relationship). But because the doctors were unschooled in psychotherapy they were unable to understand what was going on or to make proper use of it. So he decided he would have to teach them how to be therapists. That may seem to us to be going too far, but remember there were no consultation books in those days – what he really wanted to do was to teach them how to listen. He did this partly by example (giving them his full attention – no consultant had listened to GPs before) and famously by getting them to invite their problem patients back for a long interview. When they did this, they found that the multiple somatic symptoms were put aside and the patients poured out the stories of their unhappy lives – with considerable relief. Nowadays we rarely do long interviews out of choice, and Balint himself changed his mind in the 1960s, switching the focus to what could be achieved in the 'six-minute' consultation. However, as a research instrument the long interview was invaluable. Having seen the results, some of the doctors wanted to go on doing psychotherapy. This was not so easy, and some of them got into predictable difficulties. I noted with interest that one of the bravest and best of the therapist GPs was a woman, two of whose cases are discussed in depth. This now seems rather ironic in a book called *The Doctor, His Patient and the Illness*. I wonder who she was. There are 28 case histories in the book, and they give an intriguing picture of how people lived in London in the early 1950s. I have to say that their lives seem rather sad. Most of the patients are poor, and there isn't a lot to do. Rock and Roll and the Swinging Sixties have yet to arrive. The shadow of World War Two still hangs over everyone and there is a great fear of tuber-culosis. Parents are strict, and the young are sexually frustrated. Only the cinema provides some welcome entertainment.

In the later chapters of the book, Balint seems to realise that GPs can't and shouldn't try to behave like therapists. They all have their own idiosyncratic approach and can't resist giving their patients advice ('the doctor's apostolic function'). However, they do have the great advantage (or they did in the 1950s) of always being there for the patients. After facilitating some much needed emotional release, the GP could return to being your ordinary sore throat and certificate doctor – but would be ready to slip back into counsel-ling mode when the next emotional crisis came along.

Balint groups have changed quite a bit since the book was written, but it's fascinating to learn how the whole movement started. Michael Balint writes very good English (and I don't just mean for a Hungarian). Despite what you may have heard, this book is very easy to read and frequently entertaining. So I recommend that you read it again – for the first time.

DOCTORS TALKING TO PATIENTS by Patrick Byrne and Barrie Long (1976)

This modest little book is often referred to in lists of 'models of the consul-tation' served up to our registrars. But of course they don't read it. No one reads it these days, which is a shame because it was an important milestone in the development of general practice. It is also very funny and very shocking. The study which led to the book was the first attempt to record (on audio-tape) the conversations between doctors and patients in everyday surgeries. These dialogues leap off the page with all the freshness of live theatre. When you read them you may think, surely doctors don't talk in that patronising, insensitive, ignorant way nowadays? What never? I wouldn't be so sure. The big difference is that now we know we are supposed to be patient-centred, and if we do have outbreaks of naked hostility towards our patients, we don't record them for posterity.

Anyway, the doctors are not all bad. There are a few consultations in which a doctor just listens helplessly while the patient pours out her incoherent, tragic and apparently endless story. It's enough to make you weep, and not just with laughter. The authors tell us that these consultations, in which the doctor employs a 'listening and reflecting' style were as rare as hens' teeth, occurring in only 1% of their sample of over 100 GPs in the Manchester area.

Now let me tell you a little about the book's authors and how the work originated. Patrick Byrne was the first Professor of General Practice in England (he was appointed to a Chair in Manchester in 1971). One of his most valued colleagues was a university education lecturer and social scientist called Barrie Long. They both realised that there was something wrong with the standard general practice consultation, and they wanted to introduce GPs to some ideas derived from counselling and teacher training. Most of the ideas were probably Long's, but Byrne was the mover and shaker who got the project launched and financed. Legend has it that the professor was somewhat appalled by the results, and had doubts as to whether the transcripts could decently be published. In the event the book came out while Long was out of the country. On his return he was very angry, claiming that the book was '95% his' and that two-thirds of his case material had been missed out. Relationships between the co-authors were cool for a while, but they eventually made it up (see *The Life of Professor PS Byrne* by John Findlater, RCGP Publications, 1996).

So what conclusions did Barrie Long draw from all these sensational tapes? He produced the first map of the phases of the consultation, which all subsequent consultation gurus have copied with slight variations. He notes that after greeting the patient in a fairly stereotypical way, the doctor 'discovers, or attempts to discover, the reason for the patient's attendance.' Sadly, the attempt is often unsuccessful, generally because the doctor *doesn't listen*. There is also a phase called 'consideration of patient condition', which you will recognise as Neighbour's 'summarising' checkpoint. In *Doctors Talking to Patients* this one is frequently omitted, possibly because GPs then had even less time than we have now. Five minutes was the average time per patient, and after three hours or so it's not surprising that they were feeling tired and irritable. Hence the tendency to be bossy, patronising and unintentionally very funny. By analysing their behaviours, Barrie Long was able to identify four different consulting styles in the diagnostic phase, and seven in the prescribing phase. The diagnostic styles were as follows: gathering information; analysing and probing; clarifying and interpreting; listening and reflecting. Doctors tended to stick to one style throughout. As I mentioned, the reflective style (which Long clearly wished to promote) was excessively rare. What was to be done? Byrne and Long set up some training courses for GPs who wished to study and perhaps modify their consultation styles. They listened to their tapes in small groups and used role play to see how things might be done differently. It seemed possible to move a small way across the spectrum towards greater patient-centredness, but the conversion might only be temporary.

Obviously, things have changed. We now consult more skilfully and treat our patients better – thanks largely to the work of pioneers like Barrie Long, who seems to be one of the unsung heroes of general practice. So why should we read this book today? Because we are not so different from those 1970s doctors. We can still get frustrated by lack of time, annoyed by human idiosyncrasy, and impatient to reach a conclusion. We are still capable of forgetting what we have learned, temporarily discarding our humanitarian values and being beastly to our patients. These transcripts show how it happens. They also show a few doctors trying hard and achieving some rapport. And they record the struggles of the patients to cope with their lives, their feelings and their eccentric doctors in heartrending words that recall the works of Harold Pinter or Samuel Beckett.

And now it's a great pleasure to introduce Iona Heath, who will tell us about her favourite GP classic.

A FORTUNATE MAN by John Berger and Jean Mohr (1969)

If, in a lifetime, I was allowed to read only one book to help me to understand my work as a general practitioner, that book would be *A Fortunate Man*. Deciding on the book is the easy part; explaining why is perhaps more difficult. It is a collaboration between the writer John Berger and the photographer Jean Mohr, and a lasting corroboration of what Geoff Dyer has described as John Berger's unequivocal commitment to relationships of equality. There is no hierarchy of value between the text and the photographs, and each medium communicates different things to the reader. None of the photographs are duplicated in description, and none of the photographs are simple illustrations of the text. The immediacy and integrity of the photographs mean that the text can begin its exploration of what it is to be a patient and a doctor in a small and impoverished rural community at a much deeper level than would be possible without the photographs. It can move immediately behind the faces and begin to imagine what is being felt and understood in the minds of doctor and patients. In the BBC series *Another Way of Telling*, Jean Mohr explained how both he and John stayed in the house of the doctor for over a month watching his consultations and accompanying him on visits day and night. Jean shot 30 or 40 rolls of black and white film, and then they each returned to their own home and worked independently. John turned his notes into the first draft of a text, and Jean produced about 200 black and white prints. Then they met to show each other what they had done, and almost immediately it became clear that, as John Berger put it, 'Both of us have made the same mistake, we have tried to do the book all by ourselves.' And so more than half of Jean's photos were put to one side, and John sat down to rewrite his text completely. The result is text and photographs which actively augment each other, just as doctor and patient are able to do within consultations that work well.

This is a key part of the wonder – *A Fortunate Man* is a book which enacts what it portrays. The text describes the 'closely intimate recognition' required of the doctor, the 'sense of futility [that] is the essence of loneliness', and records the assertion of the doctor that 'All diffidence in my position is a fault. A form of negligence.' Neither writer nor photographer are in any sense diffident, and the result is a closely intimate recognition of what it is to work day in and day out as a general practitioner. It is to feel one's efforts to be futile but to know that just being there to acknowledge and witness the irremediable suffering of others is an essential part of the task, to experience the delight of close and generous acquaintance over many years with those whose lives are very different in almost every particular from one's own, to take pleasure in a technical task executed skilfully, and to find the courage to keep going when one feels again that constantly recurring sense of failure and inadequacy. In reading the book as a general practitioner, one has a sense of what it might be like to be the patient of a good doctor. I feel recognised and acknowledged in a way that makes me feel whole.

The continuous commitment and way of life of the doctor portrayed as *A Fortunate Man* have almost completely disappeared as doctors have slowly reduced their hours of work and their ability to provide continuing care for individual patients. Responsibilities are now shared with a skilled primary healthcare team and between general practitioners working in partnerships of increasing size, and these changes have brought undoubted benefits but also losses to both doctors and patients. Doctors are still granted very high rates of public trust, but how much of this is built on the communal memory of the dedication of a generation of fortunate men and women who worked long hours and got out of bed at night to provide continuing care for their patients? How long can trust survive within a system where doctors work in shifts and fewer and fewer people see the same doctor twice? Our current government is intent on offering patients choice, and insists that when they need a referral to hospital, patients must be offered a choice of five different providers, including at least one from the private sector. I have yet to meet a patient who is interested in this sort of choice, but I know many who would choose to see a familiar doctor when they feel ill and frightened. This is a choice which is available to fewer and fewer. Are we still fortunate?

Iona Heath

A TEXTBOOK OF FAMILY MEDICINE by Ian R McWhinney (1997)

(First edition published as *An Introduction to Family Medicine*, in 1981.)

Ian McWhinney is one of the founding fathers of the new general practice. He was born in Burnley, Lancashire in 1926, and practised as a GP in Stratford-upon-Avon before moving to Canada and becoming Professor of Family Medicine at the University of Western Ontario. I treasure the memory of hearing him give an inspiring lecture on 'The Physician as Healer' at the International Balint Congress in Oxford in 1998. The essence of that talk was that doctors have traditionally tried to practise medicine with the emotions of both doctor and patient left out, and it just doesn't work. I think the recognition of the patient as a unique individual whose thoughts, feelings and bodily sensations are indivisible is probably McWhinney's greatest contribution to primary care medicine. He has also been influential in carving a place for primary care as an academic discipline.

So let us take a look at his book. In its latest incarnation it has four sections, of which the first, on basic principles, is in my view the most important.

Part Two gives us examples of family medicine at work in five different illnesses – sore throat, headache, fatigue, hypertension and diabetes. Parts Three and Four give the impression of having been tacked on to bring the book up to date and to make sure that it is comprehensive. They include such topics as records, home care, practice management and research. They are all very brief, and are better dealt with in twenty-first-century accounts.

Part One is the golden book that contains McWhinney's magnificent, passionate and eloquent exposition of what general practice (or family medicine as they call it across the Pond) is all about. After an initial survey of our history, in Chapter Two ('Principles') he gives us his famous list of the nine things that family physicians do. (Compare the section 'Being a general practitioner' in our own dear Curriculum.) Number one lays down that our specialty is the individual person who is allowed to present us with virtually any problem he likes. Lest we get too carried away, subsequent principles remind us that we need to be aware of the community, and practise a bit of prevention. But you may be surprised to read that we also need to see our patients in their homes and that ideally we should live in the same community. Then he deals conclusively with our lurking fear that we are not as good as the real specialists, by dismissing six popular misconceptions. A good generalist, he concludes, is the equal of a good specialist in any field. Well, we knew that really, but it's nice to have a famous professor to argue the case.

Chapters Three and Four deal with illness in the community and the kind of symptoms that family doctors commonly encounter. Then the exciting Chapter Five (philosophical and scientific foundations) introduces the great paradigm change – an illness is not a disease entity, but rather it is something happening to a person whose mind and body are one and whose health is influenced by the worlds he lives in and the relationship network that surrounds (or excludes) him. There's a wonderful extract from a clinico-pathological conference on a patient who has expired from coeliac disease, in which the GP pipes up 'I feel that he died because all that he had lived for had somehow come to nothing.' The professor of medicine says 'Thank you very much' and moves on quickly, ignoring this arresting contribution completely. McWhinney tells us about Engel and his groundbreaking biopsychosocial model. Then he goes on to quote Alfred Korzybski, who in 1958 produced the stunning aphorism 'The map is not the territory.' What does this mean? Well, the map is our clinical knowledge base which tells in abstract terms what an illness will look like. But to find out what people actually experience – and give them the help they need – 'there comes a time when we have to set aside our maps and walk hand-in-hand with the patient through the territory.'

Chapter Six is devoted to an examination of illness, suffering and healing. Patients, including medics, describe their own experiences, and writers such as Jane Austen, Fyodor Dostoyevsky, John Donne and Oscar Wilde are called as witnesses. You don't find stuff like this in many textbooks of medicine. Chapter Seven follows with an examination of doctor–patient communication. We are reminded that every bodily symptom is trying to tell us something in its own language of physical sensation blended with emotion. We look at what makes a difficult patient – and a difficult doctor. Now we reach the climax of the book, in which McWhinney unveils his *'patient-centred clinical method.'* This, although obviously very innovative in its time (the 1980s) and place (North America), may not seem to us very different from our own 'consultation models' in which we listen carefully to our patient, try to notice the flags he is desperately waving to attract our attention ('cues'), and allow him to share in the subsequent decision making. But it is fascinating to see a different group of doctors in a parallel (transatlantic) universe working along similar lines to Tate, Neighbour, *et al.* The last two chapters deal with health promotion and the family. They are interesting and well written, but you will find what they have to say is already familiar.

Should we recommend this book to our students and registrars? I think we should, but if they are not very good at reading books all the way through, we can prescribe those chapters in Part One that have true classic status and make us realise important truths about ourselves and our work.

THE INNER CONSULTATION: HOW TO DEVELOP AN EFFECTIVE AND INTUITIVE CONSULTING STYLE by Roger Neighbour (1987)

The Inner Consultation was first published in 1987, so it is old enough to be considered for classic status, and has certainly earned it. Despite all of the changes that have taken place in general practice during the last 20 years, the consultation is still the jewel in our crown, and Roger's book is the one that trainers recommend and registrars read. It must be the most influential book about general practice since Balint. So how does it appear today? When did you last open it? Let's have a look.

To begin with, we have a whole clutch of what I can only call Curtain Raisers or Opening Gambits. There are two forewords, a fore-poem (by John Bunyan), a guarantee of efficacy (daring and unusual) and a special introduction to the second edition (2004). Then there is the overview, which is like the overture to an opera, in which all the themes are presented before the curtain goes up and the audience is aroused to a keen anticipation. And of course when the show starts, it's a real treat.

Roger uses a variety of methods to make his teaching appeal to both the left and the right brain. In addition to an easily flowing conversational text, we get poems, cartoons, wise and witty sayings from East and West, metaphors, fables and exercises. When it's time for a breather we get a pit stop. And threading through the book is the ongoing tutorial with the long-suffering 'Chris', to whom all this is very new. How will I remember all this? How am I going to keep my two heads from interrupting each other? What if I forget to use my clinical skills? It's nice to have someone to voice our own worries, and reassuring to have Roger as our trainer.

Shall I remind you how the book is structured? It's as simple as ABC. Section A sets out the map of the journey that is the consultation. Section B teaches us how to acquire and polish the skills that we shall need, and Section C, which is quite short, puts it all together. Again a musical metaphor occurs to me – the symphonic structure of exposition, development, recapitulation and coda. I remember that RN is a pretty good violinist.

As I read, I come across all those phrases which have entered the GP language and become part of the culture. The five checkpoints, naturally (do you remember tapping them out on the fingers of your left hand with your right index finger, and perhaps thinking 'why am I doing this?'). Incidentally, I think Roger was the first person to include safety-netting and housekeeping as essential elements of the consultation.

Then there are those two heads fighting for control of the poor little trainee's mind – symbols of the two sides of Roger and of all of us. The logical organiser and the intuitive responder, the conscious and the unconscious, the scientist and the artist, the classicist and the romantic. We realise that this is where we first read about minimal cues, interior search and the all-important 'acceptance set.' We learn to become aware of all these things and then to relax and let them just become part of the background. We are perhaps a little surprised to learn that these new skills were really there all the time – they come along with being human, if only we can relax and trust our ability to make friends with people. The Zen masters and the tennis coach knew this, and so in fact did we all. I was struck by a phrase quite near the end of Section C about the way 'the self-assertive tendency to cling on to control of the consultation begins to slip away, to be replaced by a trusting sense of coming alongside the patient . . .' I love that image of coming alongside. I don't think I have ever read that before. I have a horrible feeling that maybe I never actually read Section C at all. I can hear Roger saying 'John, John!' But then I can remind him that 'when the pupil is ready the Master will appear.'

CHAPTER 11

Best new books about general practice

PRIMARY CARE IN THE TWENTY-FIRST CENTURY by Geoff Meads (2006)

As we hurtle towards climatic catastrophe and a future that is at best uncertain, will primary care continue to exist as we know it? Surely we will need the comforting presence of the family doctor more than ever. Not to mention some basic healthcare provision for all the survivors. So here is a book called _Primary Care in the Twenty-First Century_ by Professor Geoff Meads of Warwick University, in which he surveys the different ways in which primary care is being provided (I will not use that word _delivered_) all over the world. Geoff and his team visited an amazing 33 countries in three years and came back with a fascinating report on all the different experiments going on from China to Peru, and from Finland to Thailand – not forgetting Dorset, England.

Geoff recognises six different models, of which the first three are Extended General Practice (to be found in Greece and Finland as well as Dorset), Managed Care, and the Reformed Polyclinic. In Extended General Practice (which you will greet with glad recognition) the doctors are still just about in charge, although other potential stakeholders hover like vultures. Managed Care is, of course, run by the insurance companies, whose commitment is what Geoff archly describes as 'calculative.' Polyclinics, in case you didn't know, are aggregations of specialists (including family doctors) with government support. There are also two forms of community-based clinics, one organised by government, and the other (Geoff's favourite) springing from the grassroots and owned by the people. Here the front line is staffed by nurses, and the doctors act mainly as supervisors. Finally, there is 'Franchised Outreach', which I didn't fully understand, but it seems to mean free-for-all private enterprise with nobody in charge.

So which is the best model? That seems to depend on history, politics, local traditions and resources. There is always a trade-off between personal continuing care and universal provision of basic healthcare. As we hop from one country to another and from city to village there are lots of surprises. The polyclinic with its echoes of Soviet Russia can be found in Australia as well as Chile, while managed care is popular in both Mexico and Canada. Different systems may appear in the same country. Some developments look secure, while others are more precarious. They all seem to depend on collaboration between citizens, governments and the complete spectrum of health professionals. And as Geoff Meads rightly says, it's about ethics as well as economics. Our system comes out pretty well, but will it be replaced by one of these alternatives? This book gives an excellent overview of the possibilities. My one complaint is that I would have liked a few more interviews with individual patients, doctors and nurses. Perhaps that could be a follow-up?

COMPLEXITY IN PRIMARY CARE: UNDERSTANDING ITS VALUE
by Kieran Sweeney (2006)

How much do you know about complexity? Does your brow furrow anxiously when the word is mentioned, or are you prepared to give a lucid explanation to your lovely companion at the dinner table? If the former prevails and you would like to move towards the latter, then Kieran Sweeney's new book is the one to read. You want a brief synopsis? She's nodding her head, so here goes. Kieran, who once used a modified Balint group in one of his research projects, starts off with a case. He describes how one day in the surgery he tried to apply the principles of evidence-based medicine to 85-year-old Mrs B, who has diabetes, hypertension, osteoarthritis and a few other things to boot. His worthy scientific aim was to help her to live a few more years. But Mrs B's response was 'Well, Jack's dead and the boys have gone.' This stopped Kieran dead in his tracks. He realised (I'm sure he knew anyway) that a person's life history and her feelings are just as important as her biochemistry when you are considering the kind of doctoring that she needs. The next two chapters give us a brief history of the growth of scientific medicine (heroic and positive) and the humanistic, biographical tradition in which the patient's story and her own wishes and beliefs are taken seriously. The first approach tells us the news about a population, while the second nudges us to listen to the individual, like Mrs B, and to modify our evidence-based enthusiasm accordingly. But there's a third way of looking at medical thinking, which makes use of the findings of complexity theory. Equations begin to appear on the page, but don't panic! There are only a few. The mathematicians discovered that many processes in nature have unpredictable results because small changes can have dramatic results. At first things go pear-shaped, but then the system will often settle down in a new but different stable pattern. It's all due to feedback effects and iterative processes, you see. If it's all the same to you, we'll skip the details (they're all in Chapter Five) and go on to the medical implications. Kieran argues that complex changes can result in highly beneficial results both in organisations (such as practices) and in individual consultations. The small changes are mainly people talking and listening to one another and cooperating to get things done. Given the right conditions, complex changes can take place in a system and a new way of working can emerge. Kieran gives a nice example of the way that the Brazilian government brilliantly tackled their country's AIDS crisis by ignoring the gloomy predictions of the experts, manufacturing their own drugs and recruiting the enthusiastic help of all the existing social networks. I am reminded of the way our practice tackled the demands of the QOF framework by inviting all the receptionists to join the doctors and nurses in small teams working on different parts of the project. But can complexity help us to find the right balance between the science and human understanding when we sit in the surgery with Mrs B? And is it all underpinned by mathematics? Or is complexity theory just a useful metaphor? I'll let you decide, but *Complexity* is definitely a must for your next tutorial. Not to mention that dinner companion.

FROM GENERAL PRACTICE TO PRIMARY CARE: THE INDUSTRIALISATION OF FAMILY MEDICINE by Steve Iliffe (2008)

We are all aware of seismic changes rumbling away. But what has *really* been happening to our beloved general practice in the last 10 years? Here's a book by my old friend Steve Iliffe, who was for many years a GP in north-west London, and is now a GP academic. Steve's big revelation is that general practice has been undergoing a process akin to the Industrial Revolution. We used to be allowed by the NHS to run our own little medical businesses in any way we liked so long as we didn't bring the profession into disgrace or fail to turn up when the patients needed us. But then the government decided that it needed to move into our little workshops and turn them into mechanised factories all producing the same uniform, high-quality product. Think

McDonald's hamburgers. Whichever outlet you go into, they look and taste the same, many people like them and the place is always free of infection. And they are cheap.

How was this done to general practice? You will have noticed that we have mass production methods in that we all produce non-smoking patients with low blood pressures, low HbA_{1c}s and low cholesterol levels, for which we use identical approved drugs applied in the same order of preference. We have division of labour with nurses to manage chronic diseases, the application of science (evidence-based medicine) and the use of machinery (computerised records, automatic audit). We also have incentive bonuses to encourage us, and the threat of being displaced by private providers to keep us from rebelling. We have allowed the primary care trusts to micromanage our consultations so that we keep a careful eye on all those prompts that flash up on the screen and automatically respond with a blood pressure check or a couple of depression questions or another blood test. We save the system money by obediently undertaking specialist work as well as our own (practice-based commissioning). And we have allowed our masters to persuade us that we are really only doing what we aspire to do anyway as good little professionals – that is, respect the wisdom of evidence-based medicine as handed down to us in guidelines, save the NHS money and keep the place clean.

Steve argues that much of this is good for the patients whom we serve. After all, we want to provide everyone with the same high standard of care. We want to prevent strokes and heart attacks and avoid premature deaths. But the danger is that many of the things we do best will be crowded out and given low priority. I am talking about our tradition of personal and continuous care, of relationships which provide comfort and understanding, and of a clinical method that seeks to find meaning in illness while coping with uncertainty and ambiguity. Steve acknowledges these risks but thinks that we are strong enough to prevent these assets being lost if we engage in the management process and mitigate the cruder enthusiasms of our masters. He writes very well and his grasp of the subject is impressive. The parallel with industrialisation is a brilliant insight. But I'm not convinced by his cheerful prognosis. I think he underestimates the rate at which private healthcare firms are moving in with the blatant encouragement of the government. I keep seeing visions of the Chaplin film *Modern Times*, in which the little fellow desperately tries to keep pace with a rapidly moving assembly line on which his only task is to tighten two nuts with a spanner in each hand. You may remember that Charlie ends up being dragged into the machine and carried helplessly round the huge cogwheels, still frantically wielding his spanners.

It could happen to us.

THE CHALLENGE FOR PRIMARY CARE by Nigel Starey (2003)

So what will primary care be like in, say, ten years' time? Will all the changes, the new contracts, the frenzied activities of clinical governance, polyclinics and private providers lead to a transformation of the NHS? Nigel Starey thinks that it should and it will, and tells us all about it in his difficult but fascinating book called *The Challenge for Primary Care*. He starts off by tracing the history of primary care in the NHS, and then points out how its current structure and functioning are failing to meet the needs of both providers and patients. The basic problems, if I understand him correctly, are that we are still too focused on disease instead of health promotion, the different health professionals (doctors, nurses, pharmacists, etc.) don't know how to work together or even talk to each other, and the primary care service as a whole has no effective working relationship with social services, welfare and local government. To put this right, we need to turn ourselves into an organisation where everyone works together and learns together, we need a systems approach (knowing how the different parts of the system influence one another) and we need to stop trying to fix things with short-term solutions (such as waiting-list manipulation) which only shift the burden somewhere else.

Nigel offers two alternative primary care futures for us to look at. He calls them 'caricatures', but they seem very credible possibilities to me, and both of them are a little scary. The 'Choice First' model relies on individuals taking responsibility for their own health. Everyone has a 'personal investment account', evidently a form of compulsory health insurance with a government or employer's subsidy. This needs to be topped up by additional voluntary contributions which will enable you to purchase new more expensive treatments if you so choose. If you can't afford it, that's tough. Alternatively, if you prefer a more soft-edged socialist model, there is 'The Feel Good Factor.' Here everyone is a member of the Health Bureau, whose business is the welfare of the community as a whole. Rather like a primary care trust, the Bureau makes its facilities available to everyone who needs them, and everything is state funded. But you are expected to take notice of advice about diet, smoking and other risk factors.

Both systems, we are told, have excellent quality assurance and smoothly coordinated teamwork.

Meanwhile, what has happened to the old-fashioned family doctor? Is there a place for us in this gleaming new world? Well, yes and no. All health-care team members will share the same basic training 'up to NVQ level 4 in biological science, welfare law and community development.' After that, there are opportunities for further study and specialised learning. The person who used to be the GP (that includes you and me if we agree to stay on and do some retraining) will no longer see all the babies with coughs, etc., but will become a 'clinical care director' responsible for organising the care packages for patients with complex needs. However, our diagnostic skills will still be needed from time to time. One bit of good news is that there will be no more repeat prescriptions. Medicines will be managed by a new breed of pharmacists who are trained to be managers of therapeutics rather than shopkeepers. Is this really what is going to happen? Or are we heading for a Brave New World dystopia? Predicting the future is a dangerous game, but Nigel's analysis is convincing. I think you should read his book and show it to your registrar, who might be more receptive to change than you are. On the other hand, my registrar says she likes general practice just the way it is and she loves to see babies with coughs and rashes. Oh well, it's their future and they must work it out.

MATTERS OF LIFE AND DEATH: KEY WRITINGS by Iona Heath (2008)

In my young days I used to spend time talking to patients with terminal cancer and getting myself into trouble by telling them they were going to die. But the end of out-of-hours on call and the arrival of the palliative care team have between them put an end to those conversations, which I regret. Now here is a new book by Iona Heath, which may encourage me to make the effort to get out and visit a few more deathbeds before I take to my own.

Iona tells us in *Matters of Life and Death* that she is using words as signposts to help her find her way. She has gathered together a wonderful collection of quotations from doctors, poets, philosophers and visionaries and used them as a basis for her exploration of what death truly means for patients and their family doctors.

One of the many problems I have noticed about death is that it is both certain and uncertain. As Hamlet says (if I may be allowed a quotation or two of my own):

> If it be now, 'tis not to come. If it be not to come, it will be now.
> If it be not now, yet it will come.
> The readiness is all.

The trouble is that when the time comes, few of us are ready. The patient wants to go on living, the doctor pretends that is possible, Bergman's knight offers Death a game of chess, and so on. Personally, I have always favoured sudden death, although I know it leaves the loved ones lonely. Iona quite rightly tells us that death is part of life, and by exiting suddenly we are deprived of the opportunity to end our story properly. But hey, who cares, I would say to myself, I'm out of here, I'm gone, as quick as I can. My favourite death quotation comes from Woody Allen: 'It's not that I'm afraid of death. I just don't want to be there when it happens.' But Death too has a sense of humour, and he may decide to prolong my going, in which case I shall make the best of it and try to construct a satisfying narrative of my life for the benefit of my loved ones as well as what remains of myself. Iona quotes a good deal from Samuel Beckett's wonderful short novel *Malone Dies*, and she has inspired me to start reading it again. At the beginning of his monologue, Malone announces that he is going to occupy his last hours by telling himself three stories, and then, if time permits, making an inventory of his possessions. But first he has decided to remind himself of his present state. This he thinks is probably a mistake.

Iona suggests that we use the time to explore memory, tell a story of achievement (we have all achieved something) 'and to say explicitly and repeatedly all the precious things that, too often, are said only at funerals.' In later chapters, she talks about some unsettling aspects of death and the way we regard it. What is our relationship, as we die, to all those people who have gone before us? In memory and imagination, she points out, they are always present, part of the entire human community. As we get older, more of the people we know are dead than are still alive, and that may make it easier for us to accept that we have to go, too.

But where does the genial family doctor come into all this? What has happened to Auden's endomorphic doctor who 'with a twinkle in his eye will tell me that I have to die'? Iona reminds us that as well as being able to hold the dying patient's gaze, the doctor needs to have access to both science and poetry and to have the patience to stay till the end. Are there still family doctors who can do all that? The second part of Iona's book is a reissue of her inspiring 1995 text *The Mystery of General Practice*. If the core values of general practice were threatened then, they are now bound to the railway track with the New Labour Darzi Express thundering towards them. Iona points out that the politicians and planners have completely failed to understand what general practice is about. She systematically lays bare the ways in which the ideals of the NHS have been betrayed by consumerism, greed, misconceptions about the role of health promotion, the myth of cure, and a denial of the importance of poverty and social neglect as causes of illness and despair. Finally, she reminds us why traditional general practice could remain a vitally important power for good, if only it was allowed some freedom. Our patients already know this is true, and they remind us every day.

These Key Writings include two contributions from John Berger, the man who wrote so movingly about general practice in *A Fortunate Man*. I think I'll have that book as one of my deathbed companions along with *Malone Dies*. And probably *Anna Karenina*.

BANDOLIER'S LITTLE BOOK OF MAKING SENSE OF THE MEDICAL EVIDENCE by Andrew Moore and Henry McQuay (2006)

Here is a very small book about evidence-based medicine. No, don't run away. Look how cute it is! Only 10 by 18 centimetres, with a shiny plastic cover in pale violet and a glowing magenta stripe. And here, hold it up to your nose. Doesn't it smell nice? It's called *Bandolier*, which, in case you didn't know, is a monthly bulletin on evidence-based healthcare with jokes and a human face as well as scientific rigour.

But hasn't EBM gone out of style and lost its lustre when tested in the real world? Not at all, so long as you remember that the definition must include a reference to the care of individual, idiosyncratic patients. And if you always find statistics difficult (my hand goes up), this book is the perfect antidote. Andrew and Henry are just brilliant at finding homely metaphors to explain difficult concepts. One of their major points is the importance of size in a clinical trial. The big studies win every time, especially when the intervention has only a small effect. This is illustrated by the parable of the socks. Imagine a drawer full of red and white socks. How many would you have to pull out (without looking) in order to get a matching pair? It depends on how many of each colour are in the drawer and how sure you want to be. The answer to that, of course, is 95%-confidence-interval sure. There's another good story about throwing dice to represent a trial in which each six represents a death. With small numbers of throws the statistics may 'prove' that sixes come up more often in the control group, or vice versa. We are advised not to be impressed with *P*-values, especially if they are weaker than 0.001. Confidence intervals give more information and are much more cool. So are Numbers Needed To Treat (NNT). I have always liked that concept, so I was glad to hear that a survey of Wessex GPs in 1996 showed that 35% of them understood and could explain NNT, whereas hardly any could cope with odds ratios or relative risks. What else does *Bandolier* tell us? There is an excellent chapter on clinical trials and how to tell the good from the bad and the ugly. There is also an intriguing discussion of 'placebos' and the powerful effects of apparently doing nothing. One trial showed that placebo not only relieved pain in some patients as effectively as morphine, but also lit up the same areas in the brain. How does placebo work? We still don't know. More research is needed. Further chapters deal with observational studies, adverse events, diagnostic tests and even health economics. And there's a great little coda on 'things that don't fit in easily.' *Bandolier's* new book was fun to read and I may even remember a few things. I feel less intimidated. I might even teach some of this stuff. What more could you want?

OPHTHALMOLOGY IN PRIMARY CARE by Amar Alwitry (2005)

Why do we GPs find ophthalmology such a heart-sink subject? Is it the lack of exposure in medical school? Or the soporific effect of watching hundreds of seemingly identical slides in a darkened room? Or maybe it's all psycho-logical. Eyes are so important and so vulnerable. Out vile jelly! Ugh! But wait a moment. Here is a book which is genuinely helpful, written by an author who seems to understand our predicament – Amar Alwitry, a specialist reg-istrar who enjoys teaching. The blurb on the back cover says he also writes fiction, which I guess helps him to empathise with us poor GPs. So what do you do when a guy comes in with a red eye and says everything has gone misty? Amar asks about the presenting symptoms and with a series of gentle questions guides the reader towards a diagnosis. Even more important, he tells us *how soon* the patient should be seen in the eye clinic. Is that today, tomor-row, in the next few days, 'soon via letter' or 'routine'? This is so important and to my knowledge has never been spelt out to us before. Other invaluable paragraphs cover such questions as 'What do I need to do?', 'What will the hospital do?' and 'What shall I tell the patient?' Then there are those gnomic letters from the optometrist recommending 'urgent referral.' Mr Alwitry inter-prets these and tells us how to grade their urgency. Finally, there's a section on operations and what can go wrong. All this is in the unique, concise and invaluable first part of the book. Part Two is more like a conventional text-book, but a very good one. There are chapters on anatomy and physiology and how to examine the eye. I still remember the ophthalmologist who advised our VTS registrars not to bother buying an ophthalmoscope, as even if they saw anything they would never have enough experience to interpret it. We didn't know whether to feel excused or deeply offended. Amar, on the other hand, pays us the compliment of expecting us to have the instrument to hand and to want to know how best to use it. The rest of the book goes through all the eye problems you are likely to meet, including cataracts, detachments, glaucoma, retinopathy and age-related macular degeneration, both the wet and the dry. Everything in Part One is comfortingly cross-indexed with the detailed information in Part Two. This is a great book to have on your desk. But don't put it in the library, or it will vanish.

DIFFERENTIAL DIAGNOSIS IN DERMATOLOGY by Richard Ashton and Barbara Leppard (2004)

How do you rate yourself as a dermatologist? My own confidence rating has been flatlining since I was a student. I never seem to get any better at identifying rashes, and that is despite going to countless lectures, and watching what seem to be the same slideshows year after year. The only skin disorders I can reliably diagnose are those that I have had myself. However, that is now all about to change, thanks to a wonderful new book called *Differential Diagnosis in Dermatology* by Richard Ashton and Barbara Leppard. It's a chunky oblong tome weighing in at just over a kilogram, and it now sits in the place of honour beside my computer ready to guide me to the correct diagnosis. Why is it so good? Well, the first thing to say is that the pictures are outstanding – pin sharp, in natural colour, and almost three-dimensional in their ability to reproduce the real thing. Finding the picture you want is also easy. Each chapter deals with a different region, starting with the hairy scalp and working down via face, trunk and limbs to hands, feet and nails, not forgetting to visit the boggy folds and crevices on the way down. Each chapter also has clear algorithms to guide you to the right page, when with a cry of delight you can show the patient his identical skin twin. Furthermore, this new edition includes concise and helpful paragraphs on treatment, so therapeutic action follows swiftly in the wake of diagnostic precision. The book is also enjoyable to browse through, although there is a risk of finding pictures of one's own lumps and blemishes, previously ignored. I now know that I have lichen planus of the fingernails, for instance. But no matter, it's quite harmless (unless a complication called pterygium develops, but I am not going to worry about that, and neither should you). Please take two extra copies, as your registrar will need one, and your partners will steal the other.

CHAPTER 12

Consultation and communication

COMMUNICATION SKILLS THAT HEAL by Barry Bub (2006)

Some of you may be feeling that you are already up to here in books on communication skills. But fear not. All the ones in this section of the Green Bookshop are easy to read and have something new and intriguing to say. First of all, we have one called *Communication Skills That Heal*, by Barry Bub MD, whom you will probably not have encountered before. Barry was a family doctor in the USA for 30 years, before giving it up to devote his time to psychotherapy, teaching, running workshops and training as a chaplain. He is married to Goldie, who is a rabbi. A rabbi's wife is called a rebbetzin, so that makes Barry a hubbatzin. I wanted to share that with you. You might expect that Barry's approach to the consultation would be strongly flavoured with Jewish wisdom and humour, and you would be right. Suspicious at first, I gradually warmed to the hubbatzin's friendly and engaging manner and began underlining things that I thought were insightful (always a good sign with me). In Chapter One he talks about communications that wound rather than heal, and how easy it is to deliver them. In my surgery, a baby started screaming miserably when his father woke him up and pulled him out of the pram so that I could examine him. I nearly said (because I was feeling a bit grumpy) 'You'd have done better to stay at home and let him sleep' but, remembering Barry's advice, I stopped myself. Dr Bub goes on to remind us that the healing process can be painful, especially if you try to avoid the difficult parts, like experiencing grief. He advises doctors to put details of patients' interests and relationships in the case notes so that they become 'whole' human beings. He recommends the opening gambit of 'How are you?' rather than 'How is the illness?' OK, you have heard some of this before, but believe me, it does no harm to be reminded. And there are lots of nice little stories and dialogues illustrating the main text. A series of chapter headings anticipate the objections to studying the art of listening seriously ('But there's no time . . .' and 'But listening is so passive . . .'). There's a lovely chapter on 'laments', which refers the reader back to the Old Testament books of Lamentations, Job and the Psalms. We learn that many patients feel better when their laments are heard and validated. But if you want them to heal and stop *kvetching*, Barry says, you must help them to experience some real emotion. There are chapters about psychotherapy (Barry favours Gestalt, so if you never really understood what that is (join the club), here's a chance to find out). Then you can experiment with getting the patient to address the empty chair that represents her errant daughter. Or challenge a patient to a pillow fight. I could go on and on – but here, take a copy and read it for yourself. Enjoy.

LISTENING AS WORK IN PRIMARY CARE by Simon Cocksedge (2005)

Simon takes the view that listening is an essential part of the work that GPs do, and not just a tedious process that has to be gone through in order to extract the diagnosis. Simon conducted qualitative interviews with 23 experienced GPs in the Derbyshire Peak District. His book consists largely of extracts of what the doctors said about their listening, held together with some discussion of the issues by the author. The first point on which they are all agreed is that listening is part of the service we give to patients, part of our legitimate work, and something of which we can be proud. Listening is the basis for 'discovering why the patient has come', and if we interrupt with too many closed questions we shall fail to discover. When the patient gives a cue that there is something else on her mind, we can choose to ignore it or we can embark on a little 'listening loop', which Simon compares graphically to a sort of railway branch line. The loop, whose destination may not be strictly medical, may later rejoin the main line or it may wander off to a completely different destination. If we can cope with a few of these Shandeian digressions, so much the better, say I, although they can play havoc with your railway timetable. The doctors go on to discuss the way in which a succession of listening sessions is used to build up an ongoing relationship. This can be used for a bit of one-off pastoral counselling ('You're the only person I can talk to, doctor'), or the doctor can use regular listening sessions as a means of support or 'holding' for those patients who need it. Can there be too much listening? Well, yes, because we have to have a home life, if only to go and listen to what sort of day the spouse has had. So the doctors talk about the limits they have to use to protect their personal boundaries from incursion by patients who might get a bit too friendly, or take up too many appointments, or expect some therapeutic listening in the park or the supermarket when the good doctor is trying to concentrate on jogging or shopping. This is an absorbing, thoughtful book. The doctors' voices come off the page very vividly, and we can all share their pleasure in the work, as well as their concerns. The final chapter rounds up all of the book's themes and explores a few of the issues that arise from them. I think Simon is absolutely right to point out that the listening work that we do is undervalued by the experts (although not by the patients). So-called 'ordinary GP care' is something extra-ordinary that we should be careful not to lose.

THE NAKED CONSULTATION by Liz Moulton (2007)

Are you looking for a good, short, entertaining basic consultation book for your trainees? I know, I know, you have a shelf-ful of them already, but I promise you this one is worthy of your attention even if you have read all the others (which, to be brutally honest, you haven't). Liz Moulton is a GP educator and former Course Organiser in Yorkshire. So tell us, Liz, why *naked*? It's a catchy title reminding me of Kafka's *Country Doctor* who was stripped of his clothes and bundled into bed with his patient to continue a rather dysfunctional consultation. Well, we can all feel a bit exposed in the consulting room and, as Liz points out, we may be in special need of assistance when we are no longer beginners but could do with a little revision. She has a direct, very readable style, and in no time at all we are off on a tour of all the great consultation models, from Budapest to Calgary by way of Watford and Hemel Hempstead. The ground plan of Part One of the book is the Neighbourhood Way, and all the familiar fingerposts are revisited – but with a difference. Liz draws inspiration from a range of other communication experts, including Michael Balint, Carl Rogers, Eric Berne, John Launer and whoever invented neurolinguistic programming. There are useful tips on getting the most out of the golden moment when the patient comes through the door (try saying nothing), and coping with the problem of time. The second section is devoted to learning and personal development and is a useful summary. MRCGP candidates might find it a little frustrating that there is a whole chapter on the old video exam but nothing about the assessments and tests for the nMRCGP. Perhaps that will come in the second edition. Meanwhile this is a readable stimulating book which deserves a prominent place in your Consultation Collection.

BEHIND THE CONSULTATION by André Matalon and Stanley Rabin (2007)

Wouldn't it be nice to be able to talk about your difficult patients to a friend who can really understand? Here is a book by two Israeli clinicians who have been sharing their difficult consultations with each other for a number of years. André Matalon is a GP and his pal Stanley Rabin is a psychologist, and the two of them have written a book called *Behind the Consultation* in which they show us the benefits of their friendship and collaboration. You might think that their patients would be very different, but they are not. Both authors have been in practice for many years and they believe in continuity. And both can be deeply affected by the emotions that some of their patients evoke in them. They are especially troubled by the patients who remind them in some way of themselves. A troubled young man who needs his therapist to be a father reminds Stanley how he misses his own father whom he left behind in South Africa. An attractive young woman who tells him about her secret lover makes him fear that he is experiencing vicarious excitement. Meanwhile André, the GP, feels angry and frustrated with a depressed old man who reminds him of his need, since the age of eight, to be a doctor for his depressed mother. Then there are the patients who seem to pick you out to be the only recipient of stories of suffering that perhaps you would rather not hear because they remind you of your own losses. Other patients seem to make us identify so closely with them that our feelings seem 'unprofessional.' We need to unburden ourselves, too, with someone who can help us to clarify our thinking. At the end of each case history the two friends write a response to each other's stories. This gives the reader a real sense of the warmth of their friendship and their mutual understanding. The replies offer reassurance but also fresh insights, and always the feeling that 'I've been there too.' As a postscript, a friend and colleague, Dr Ben Maoz, adds another layer of reflection. I can recommend this book to anyone who has ever lost sleep over their relationship with a patient.

NARRATIVE-BASED PRIMARY CARE by John Launer (2002)

I have been hearing about narrative medicine for some years without really understanding what it means. Now, thanks to John Launer, I think I am at least beginning to grasp the idea. Whether I shall ever be able to practise it is another matter – but hey, why not?

So what is it about? We all know that patients have stories to tell, if only we would lower the hands that hover restlessly over the keyboard and just listen to them. But the patient's personal version of what happened (and why) may be at odds with the doctor's medical 'facts.' Obviously the doctor is the one who knows what he's talking about. Or is he? Postmodernism tells us rather worryingly that our story is not necessarily any more true than that of the patient. It's just different. Our medical account may be accepted by all the evidence-based gurus today, but in 10 years' time it could look very quaint and out of date. So what should doctor and patient do about their stories? According to narrative medicine, they should collaborate, like a pair of scriptwriters, in producing a really good story, which will be aesthetically satisfying and also helpful to the patient. For example, a patient with a story about throat pain due to heart disease may collaborate with a skilled practice nurse to produce a version in which anxiety about heart disease is dealt with by looking at the risk factors, and the throat is appeased by a few simple remedies.

The first part of the book deals with 'practice' and shows us the narrative doctor and nurse at work. I was particularly struck by the way they listen very carefully to the patient's actual words. If the patient says that his five problems are not connected, the doctor simply accepts this as true. She just asks for the most important one and pursues that to begin with. A lot of the techniques for encouraging the patient's thoughts to flow are derived from family therapy, which, John tells us, has become increasingly narrative in direction. In Chapter Two ('Concepts') we are introduced to the six C's, which begin with Conversation and Curiosity (very important). We then go on to Circularity, Contexts and Co-creation (of stories), but we end with Caution. Don't be too postmodern too quickly, Dr Launer warns, especially if your patient has clearly suffered a major blow such as stroke or a heart attack. I am sure this is good advice, although accounts of how and why the disaster happened may well become the material for a good story afterwards. Part One deals with lots of other interesting topics, including helping narratives to flow, mental health problems and, of course, families. Part Two describes the education and training in narrative medicine which goes on at the Tavistock Clinic in London. Part Three deals with theory and compares the narrative approach with earlier models of 'The Consultation.' We take a searching look at the Patient-Centred Model and discover that from the narrative point of view it is a bit hung up on old-fashioned objectivity. Sure, we must find out what the patient thinks, but he may not really know himself until he has talked about it with a practitioner who listens to his words and asks a few helpful questions. Next we examine the Balint tradition, which also values attentive listening to the patient's story. John has a number of criticisms of the Balint philosophy with which I disagree. But as a Balint disciple of many years' standing I would, wouldn't I? Clearly he and I will have to sort all this out over a few drinks.

Meanwhile I shall certainly try out some of the intriguing and challenging ideas of narrative-based medicine, and you will want to as well when you have read this book. John Launer writes with great clarity and has the enviable ability to make difficult concepts look simple. He also has a great story to tell.

CHAPTER 13

Education for primary care

Here is a short selection of the books on GP education that have impressed us in the last seven years. They comprise a two-volume textbook, a condensed Curriculum, a brilliant introduction to academic general practice, and a guide to blending medicine and the arts in the classroom.

THE OXFORD TEXTBOOK OF PRIMARY MEDICAL CARE
Chief Editor: Roger Jones (2004)

Do you need something really impressive to grace the shelves of the practice library? Look no further. Ladies and gentlemen – I am about to show you the biggest book that the Green Bookshop has ever offered to its customers. Let us first of all appraise its physical presence. The book weighs in at four kilograms. Its two handsome blue volumes contain 1300 pages and about 1.5 million words provided by no less than 400 contributors from all over the world (but chiefly the UK, North America and the Netherlands). Inside the back cover of Volume Two there is also a CD-ROM. This colossal piece of work is the new *Oxford Textbook of Primary Medical Care*. It has a serious claim to contain everything you could possibly want or need to know about general practice. Have the 400 authors pulled it off? Let us have a look.

Volume One is subtitled 'Principles and Concepts', and its chapters add up to a grand and comprehensive survey of the world of primary care medicine. Everything you would expect to find in a major reference work is here. I can't possibly mention every topic, but if you or your registrar were looking for accounts of the history of the general practitioner, or the state of primary care in different countries around the world, or why people go to the doctor, or what goes on in the consultation, you would find it all within. There are also, as you would hope and expect, sections on health promotion, research, education and even practice management. Are they authoritative and well written? Well, I haven't read them all but I have dipped into many chapters on your behalf, and I am impressed.

When faced with an encyclopaedic book like this I tend to head first for the subjects I know something about, to see if I agree with the authors. So I read and enjoyed all the seven essays on the consultation. The ideas were mostly familiar, but I found the presentations refreshing, and it was interesting to learn about the patient-centred method, which is the North American version of how to do a good consultation. I thought the first chapter, on the patient–doctor relationship, by Anne Louise Kinmonth and Moira Stewart was an excellent introduction, and I was intrigued to learn that there were not one but two schools of Ancient Greek Medicine. The School of Cos (chaired by Hippocrates) favoured the whole patient approach, whereas the physicians of Cnidus were more interested in understanding the disease process. It occurred to me that medicine remains divided by the deep split between these approaches, and indeed the very book I was reading reflects the division by its separation into two volumes. I shall return to this problem later on. Skipping along to the end of Volume One, I especially liked Wayne Weston's chapter on the ethical perspectives in the doctor–patient relationship. He talks about the unconscious factors that lead patients to treat us like their parents. He doesn't mention Balint, but he does produce a revealing quotation from Anna Freud ('The patient . . . will do his best to push you into a position of parental authority'). He also introduces an American writer called Anatole Broyard, who wrote about his experience as a cancer patient:

> I wouldn't demand a lot of my doctor's time. I just wish he would brood on my situation for perhaps five minutes, that he would give me his whole mind just once . . . I'd like my doctor to scan me, to grope for my spirit as well as my prostate. Without such recognition, I am nothing but my illness.

Moving on to the Cnidian Volume Two, we find a very thorough, very comprehensive but rather conventional textbook. All of the systems (cardiovascular, respiratory, digestive, etc.) are there, and all of their disorders are described in the traditional way. The specialties of the eye, ear, nose, throat and skin (which we never managed to grasp in medical school) are set forth once again. The special people – women, children, the old and the psychologically disturbed

– are all represented. In terms of treatment, we are told what works, what is supported by the evidence and what is more doubtful. I looked up a dozen topics about which I had Doctors' Educational Needs. I found the appropriate sections well written, helpful and well referenced. I very much liked the chapter by Joe Kai on 'The Approach to the Sick Infant', and would recommend it to every new GP registrar. Do I have any criticisms? One problem with a work like this is that bits of it will inevitably have become out of date by the time the book is published. I noted that we are no longer likely to recommend women to take HRT for up to 20 years, and we have definitely decided that it doesn't do the heart any favours. A more curious anomaly arises from the international mix of authors. I was surprised to find that the American authors of the chapter on 'Childhood Respiratory Infections' were very concerned to identify the 'strep throat' and treat it vigorously with penicillin in order to avoid rheumatic fever and glomerulonephritis. I thought we now had evidence that this was completely unnecessary. And indeed the counterbalancing European view is presented in a different part of the book by Professor Verheij of Utrecht (whom God preserve).

Fascinated and completely hooked, I continued browsing. The *Oxford Textbook* is very seductive, and sampling one chapter quickly leads to another and another. My eye was caught by a chapter on neck pain. How, I wondered, would the authors deal with something common, chronic and impossible to understand or treat? Everything diagnostic and therapeutic was presented and evaluated. But something was missing. There was no account of the way a GP has to spend time just sitting and listening and sharing the pain. It occurred to me that all this sort of thing was in the first volume in a general way, but that I could do with something more holistic and Hippocratic in the disease management chapters, too. Whatever the disease or the symptoms, we need to feel the presence of the GP as a witness and a steadfast companion in times of suffering. We need to know how the patient feels. We need to know how the patient's pain makes the doctor feel. We need some more medical humanity with our special subjects. And then I began to think of all the problems that patients bring us which are not really illnesses at all. Shouldn't we have chapters on problems with husbands, worries about children, disputes at work requiring prolonged sick certification, housing problems, noisy neighbours, requests for impossible letters, refugee problems and language problems? But maybe that would be a different kind of book – perhaps a 'Companion' to Primary Care rather than a Compendium. Meanwhile, despite these niggles, I do think this book is a great achievement and a superb work of reference.

The price may seem a bit steep at £295, but your practice's substantial income from Quality Street will absorb that in no time.

And so to the Curriculum, which is represented by:

THE CONDENSED CURRICULUM GUIDE by Ben Riley, Jayne Haynes and Steve Field (2008)

In 1972, the Royal College of General Practitioners published a book called *The Future General Practitioner: Learning and Teaching*. Its aim was to set out the curriculum for a revived and reinvented general practice. We were now a specialty in our own right and our trainees were going to receive a proper education from professionally trained teachers. That education would embrace not just conventional medicine, but also the comprehensive care and understanding of the patient in physical, psychological and social terms. The book was regarded as a difficult read, but it set the agenda for training and defined the way we thought of ourselves.

Now, 35 years later, we have a new book destined to become the sacred text of GP education for the next few decades. Ben Riley, Jayne Haynes and Steve Field have pored over the new curriculum with its 32 statements, 1350 learning outcomes and 500 pages and brought forth *The Condensed Curriculum Guide*. Do we need a guide as well as a condensation? We certainly do, because the curriculum has a complex and cunning structure as well as a vocabulary of its own, and these can be quite perplexing. That word reminds me of the twelfth-century Jewish scholar Moses Maimonides who wrote a book called *A Guide for the Perplexed* for the benefit of those struggling to understand God, the Universe and Everything. You will be interested to know that he also practised as a doctor. But back to the curriculum. As well as having 32 statements, it speaks of the six core competences or domains, which provide a kind of framework that reminds us of our overall aims and intentions in learning so much detailed knowledge. So we have *primary care management* (1) and *specific problem-solving skills* (3), but we also have *person-centred care* (2) and *a holistic approach* (6). Each domain is divided up into competencies (not the same as *competences*, but try not to let this bother you), and these in turn are made up of a number of learning outcomes which can be *knowledge, skills* or *attitudes*. Full of admiration as I am, I have to ask, is this Linnaean taxonomy entirely necessary?

And having grasped the structure and content of the curriculum, what should we do with it? Here the Guide part of the book comes into its own. There are excellent chapters on how GPs learn and how they can teach. The material used is probably familiar from the other GP education books pub-lished in the last 10 years, but it does no harm to have it all summarised and matched to the curriculum. There is also a helpful chapter on the nMRCGP and how its multifarious assessments are designed to capture the content of the curriculum. Finally, we come to the 32 statements themselves, in sum-marised form. These basically tell you in detail everything you have to know and do to be an effective GP. It may not be rocket science, but it is still pretty impressive. I'm reminded of the parson in Oliver Goldsmith's poem *The Deserted Village*:

> Amaz'd the gazing rustics gathered round;
> And still the wonder grew
> That one small head could carry all he knew.

In this section the bare statements of the curriculum are first condensed and then expanded by the generous provision of *tips*. These are little commentar-ies on how to learn something – look it up, keep a diary, shadow a palliative care nurse, attend a clinic, do an audit. These tips are genuinely educational and bring us to the underlying question of how we are to use the curriculum. Should we teach it systematically (this week dermatology, next week palli-ative care, etc.) or will this do our little heads in? What's wrong with the good old apprenticeship model? Don't we learn best from what we need at the time? But how can we be sure to cover everything that way? This debate will run and run, and the Condensed Curriculum will happily be there as a companion and Guide for the Perplexed. And do have a look at *The Future General Practitioner*. You'll find it gathering dust on a remote upper shelf in the practice library.

PRIMARY HEALTH CARE: THEORY AND PRACTICE
by Trisha Greenhalgh (2007)

I spend Wednesday afternoons in the ground-floor postgraduate centre at the Whittington, having fun doing postgraduate education with the GP trainees. Several floors above us, in her department, is Professor Trisha Greenhalgh, who teaches and researches academic primary care. Occasionally our paths cross in the corridor or car park and she gives me a fleeting half smile as one who thinks 'I know him from somewhere but can't place him.' I'd love to stop her for a chat, but she must be incredibly busy, so I don't dare. Perhaps a review of her latest book will help to arouse her curiosity. And what a book!

It's called *Primary Health Care: Theory and Practice*, and it's very readable as well as awe-inspiringly scholarly. Although she works in her ivory tower, the professor is also very well grounded in her down-to-earth life as a part-time GP and full-time working mother. The book, she tells us, is intended for aspiring academics in the field, but also for reflective practitioners (among whom we include ourselves, don't we?) and anyone else who is interested. Trisha emphasises the importance of multi-disciplinary working, but points out that she wrote this book all by herself. That personal touch is very important, and the 'I' pronoun helps us to feel as if we are her students and she is talking to *us*.

In her preface, she pays tribute to some legendary predecessors in the serious study of our work, including Julian Tudor Hart, Ian McWhinney and Michael Balint. Then she gives us some definitions of primary healthcare, but admits that they fail to convey the 'mixture of elation and terror' which she felt on assuming responsibility for her first list of 2000 people. We probably have a rough idea of what primary care is, but what is meant by academic study? Trisha maintains that there is 'nothing so practical as a good theory' when you are trying to understand something. And primary care now has at its disposal an impressive array of 'ologies' which can be deployed by the eager young researcher. They include the biomedical sciences (now with evidence-based medicine), but also the more elusive disciplines such as psychology, sociology, anthropology and philosophy.

Now we are ready to learn about research methods, both qualitative and quantitative, and how and where to deploy them. After that we move into the familiar territory of the consulting room, with chapters on the patient, the clinician and their interaction. Again, lots of approaches are available, depending on which aspect you want to study. You may at heart be a rationalist, for whom accurate diagnosis and treatment is the goal. Or you may be a soft-centred old humanist who likes to listen to her patients' stories and wonder what they mean. You may even be a nurse practitioner with a perspective of her own. However, as Trisha keeps reminding us, we need to be adept in a number of different styles depending on the patient's needs. The book winds towards its close with excellent chapters on the population, the community, the family (or lack of it) and the difficult task of improving the lives of our many patients with complex multi-illness problems. Finally we take a look at quality – what it means and how you recognise it. I should add that each chapter has a stack of interesting-looking references.

I really enjoyed this book, and although it's academic I seemed to understand most of it, which is a tribute to the author. However, I do have one big question. Although Balint and McWhinney and the 'patient-centred method' are given their due, there is no mention of Roger Neighbour or Peter Tate or any of the other modern gurus of the consultation. Not that I'm complaining, you understand, because there is no shortage of books on the consultation, not to mention the curriculum and how to pass the new MRCGP. But I wonder if there is some sort of gulf or Grand Canyon separating academic primary care from learning to be a primary care doctor. Perhaps this would be a subject to broach next time that elusive professor hurries past me in the corridor with her enigmatic smile.

THE ARTS IN MEDICAL EDUCATION: A PRACTICAL GUIDE by Elaine Powley and Roger Higson (2005)

Here's a book after my own heart. It is full of enthusiasm for the subject and has lots of practical suggestions for introducing novels, poems, pictures, drama and even music into the VTS curriculum. It's written by two experienced medical educators, Elaine Powley and Roger Higson, both of whom have been course organisers, which always gives people street cred in the Green Bookshop. They are ably assisted by David Powley, who contributes the chapter on drama, and George Taylor, who provides a good introduction.

In their opening chapter, Elaine and Roger say that the arts can create a bridge between medical science and human experience. In Chapter Two they offer some very practical instructions on building those bridges. You want to do an arts session with medics? Start with a clear aim (a subject such as breaking bad news) and then look for an artistic resource which 'will catch the drama of the moment.' It can be a painting, a poem, a film extract, a mini-drama or even an outing to the country. Then give the group time to respond, explore their responses and encourage them to reflect on what they have learned in crossing the bridge.

After this outline of the method (illustrated with an example using a film extract), there is a chapter each on stories, poetry, music, visual arts, trips to parks and galleries and the use of drama. There are lots of examples, some familiar, others new and intriguing. I should add that not only is this book beautifully illustrated with excellent colour reproductions, but also it has a CD with music examples coyly peeping out of the inside of the front cover. I played this through at once and found lots of favourite classical pieces. It was just a little frustrating not to be told who the artists were (and also not to be able to hear the works in full). Happily I was led back to my own CD collection and had a lovely evening listening to Mozart symphonies and Beethoven's opus 130 quartet in B flat, the one with that anguished *cavatina*, followed by a dancing allegro or the Grosse Fugue, depending on your mood.

Now I am looking forward to trying some of the many imaginative exercises which the book generously offered, and when you have read it I am sure you will want to do the same. I especially liked the idea of starting with a case history or a hospital letter and re-imagining it from the patient's point of view. And the drama games, starting with the one where you sit in a circle, catch someone's eye and then meet briefly in the middle with a word, a gesture or a touch before quickly exchanging seats . . .

A lovely book, a touch expensive at £40, but you do get the CD and the pictures included. Damn the expense. Lose it in the practice/library/departmental budget.

CHAPTER 14

Psychiatry, psychology and a bit of philosophy

Let's move over to the Mental Health Section. GPs are always interested in the mind because patients' personalities are so much in evidence in our surgeries. We are often told that an amazingly high proportion of our consultations are about people's mental health problems. Some of the experts tell us that we continually fail to diagnose 'depression.' It is suggested that depressed patients deceive us by presenting their depressive illness under the guise of physical symptoms. We need to teach them how to convert their bodily symptoms back into emotions, so that we can give them antidepressants. And while we are trying to digest all this, along comes Professor McWhinney to remind us that the mind and the body are all one. This is confusing, so obviously we will be in need of some good books about the science and medicine of mind. To which I will add a pinch of philosophy.

Let's start with:

BEYOND DEPRESSION: A NEW APPROACH TO UNDERSTANDING AND MANAGEMENT by Christopher Dowrick (2004)

I think this is a brilliant book. Christopher Dowrick is Professor of Primary Care at Liverpool University. I have not had the pleasure of meeting him but, having read his book, I know that he is married with six children, enjoys reading literature and philosophy and plays golf rather badly. I also deduce that as well as being a much published academic he is a real GP who has known some of his patients for decades. Christopher's book invites us to challenge the whole idea of 'depression' as an illness that needs medical treatment. His starting point is Robert Burton's *Anatomy of Melancholia,* which provides a long-winded but comprehensive and still relevant account of the condition. Having introduced us to this great work with some tempting quotations, the Professor then provides a brief map of the journey on which he is about to take us. He begins (in Chapter Two) by putting the case for our present-day disease-centred approach to depression, including the definitions, the epidemiology and the treatment. Then, in Chapter Three, he dons wig and gown, becomes counsel for the prosecution and starts to undermine everything we have been taught. We learn that psychiatrists themselves can't agree on the definition of depression. The symptoms seem to overlap confusingly not only with those of other kinds of mental suffering, such as anxiety, but also with those of back pain, heart disease, unexplained physical symptoms and just plain old social problems. A cool critical eye is cast on the research evidence for depression as a biological disorder. All right, maybe it's not so simple, but antidepressants are very effective, aren't they? Well, maybe not. There's a big placebo effect, and for some reason it's increasing. Another intriguing research finding is that patients whose 'depression' is not detected by their hapless GP actually fare better than those whom he diagnoses and treats with tablets.

In Chapter Four the prosecutor really gets going. He puts it to us that there are all sorts of vested interests involved in persuading us that depression is a disease. The drug firms have joyfully seized on it as a marketing opportunity. Psychiatrists win more respect from physicians by using a biochemical approach and talking like proper doctors. Academics retain their jobs by writing lots of papers. Even we GPs feel better if we can solve those complicated life problems we don't really want to hear about by prescribing a single daily tablet.

But the downside of all this dubious medicalisation of human unhappiness has to be measured in side-effects, lifelong medication and sheer ineffectiveness. When I look at my patients who are taking an antidepressant, I find that most of them have been on it for years and they are still miserable. There must be a better way, and Christopher has some inspiring suggestions. In Chapter Five ('Broadening the Mind') he takes us on a tour of anthropological, linguistic, philosophical and literary contributions to the investigation of sadness and depression. We learn about the medieval sin (or 'synne') of *accidie,* and the poetic state of *ennui,* both of which seem to describe a despondent feeling that life is pointless and not worth getting out of bed for. Then there's the Buddhist concept of *Dukkha,* which reminds us that to live is to suffer, and that any happiness we achieve will, like life itself, be transient. I think we all know the pithy modern summary of that one.

So what is to be done to help our unhappy patients if their misery cannot be charmed away with the magic of Prozac or even venlafaxine? I think we all have some idea of the answer to that one, too, but in his final chapters Christopher describes it beautifully. With illustrations from literature and from his own patients, he reminds us that to cope with life we have to have a sense of ourselves as real and enduring. We need to engage with life in the community so that we have a network of people whose friendship supports and renews us. We need to feel that our life has some meaning if it is to have any sweetness. Christopher warns against too much introspection, but warmly recommends good conversation with your doctor. He reminds us how important it is to listen and share the feelings. But he also recommends a more active approach, with suggestions about getting more involved with life (like taking up a hobby, doing voluntary work or falling in love). And patients also need our help to tell a better story about themselves. I really enjoyed this book. It is controversial and provocative but also full of old-fashioned wisdom, and if you like your wisdom to be evidence based, there are plenty of references. I think it deserves to become a classic.

MIND FROM BRAIN by Kenneth Sanders (2006)

Kenneth Sanders, the author of this book, was a GP for 35 years and a psychoanalyst in his spare time. You may like to know that he is also my elder brother. Is this declaring an interest? I should say so. Now as brother Ken listened to his GP patients, he found that the psychoanalytical model of the mind offered him a way of making sense of their stories and their lives. He starts the book by bringing us up to date on the work of some of Freud's successors in the last 60 years. We have all heard of 'the inner child', but today's analysts see the mind populated by a whole family, including mother, father, brothers and sisters. The inner mother feeds and nourishes us and is in turn revived and refreshed by her relationship with the internal father. Unfortunately, we get jealous of our inner parents' intimacy and try to disrupt it, with potentially disastrous consequences for our health and happiness.

During his years in practice Kenneth was exposed, just as we are, to hundreds of patients coming into the surgery with inexplicable symptoms. His psychoanalytical training and his insatiable curiosity led him to ask them about their childhood and their families. They were nearly always ready to oblige, and he collected a compendium of moving little tales of lives lived with quiet or sometimes noisy desperation. In return he interpreted their stories and symptoms in terms of the 'inner family.' Some patients were intrigued and, although most were sceptical, they often came back to hear the same story again.

How was this helpful? To find the answer we can turn to another psycho-analytical idea – the concept of the mother as a 'container', holding her baby and accepting all the negative emotions that he or she needs to get rid of. Her state of mind when she does this has been called 'the maternal reverie.' Being a good container is also what we do as doctors when we just listen and give our undivided attention for 10 or 15 minutes. The baby discharges its disagreeable stuff (faecal and emotional) and gets a clean nappy and a hug in return. The patient gets the same service metaphorically. It works, so long as we can avoid feeling smothered in emotional excrement. If that happens we may need a bit of a clean-up ourselves.

Mind from Brain consists of a series of clinical vignettes based on the doctor's records and covering all the Seven Ages of Man and Woman, from tiny babies to half-crazed old grannies. Each is followed by a brief retrospective psychoanalytical commentary. The clinical stories (one of which has pictures) are framed by two chapters which explain the theory briefly and with clarity. There is a helpful glossary of terms like 'counter-transference' at the end. Whatever you think about the internal family, this book will grab your attention and refresh your interest in patients' lives and loves.

MENTAL HEALTH IN PRIMARY CARE: A NEW APPROACH edited by Andrew Elder and Jeremy Holmes (2002)

Before I stopped going to dinner parties I would sometimes be asked by my neighbour if it was true that 70% of GP consultations were for psychological problems. Well, I would say, it all depends what you mean by 'psychological' – everyone is human and has thoughts and feelings which may distress them or make them ill. The brain is an organ like any other; and it drips emotions in the same way that a kidney produces urine. Mind and body are indivisible, and we deal with whole people. Then a troubled look would come into my companion's beautiful eyes and she would say 'But surely some of them are really mentally ill? And is it true you only have 10 minutes?'

Well, we all know it's not easy to deal with pain, fear, distress, possible cancer and a touch of madness in the space of 10 minutes. A little help is always welcome, and here it comes in the compact shape and purple cover of *Mental Health in Primary Care: a new approach*. The editors, Andrew Elder (GP) and Jeremy Holmes (consultant psychotherapist) have assembled a brilliant team of 26 contributors who take us all the way from the first heart-sinking moment in the surgery to the gratefully received evidence-based advice of the specialist.

The book starts with some accounts of what it's like to listen to strange thoughts and disturbed feelings in the surgery. We consider the relationship between psyche and soma and try to put them back together. We examine the significance of time in the lives of patients and doctors, and we explore the ways in which our mental health services might become more humane and more effective. Poets are called in to give their valuable testimony. The second part looks at 'difficult patients' and discusses how GPs can help themselves to contain and to understand all the pain, distress and uncertainty that patients bring. Can we avoid being difficult doctors and still escape brain death by spontaneous combustion? We need to feel loved and valued ourselves, both at home and in the practice, and it's good to be able to talk about our work with colleagues, individually or in a group. The third part examines what goes on in the practice outside the 10-minute consultation. We can use ideas from family (systems) therapy which will expand our repertoire, and the presence of a counsellor or therapist can help both doctors and patients in many different ways. Indeed, the practice as a whole can be 'a community of listeners', helping to make distressed patients feel that they have come to a place where they are accepted and understood.

The final part of the book is written by mental health specialists. It is really a short textbook of psychiatry for GPs, with chapters on selected common illnesses (e.g. postnatal depression, eating disorders, substance abuse) and on treatment methods (medical and psychological). The tone is now prescriptive rather than reflective, and the editors are apologetic about this in their introduction. I get the impression that they tried to get the specialists to tell us a little about how the work affects them as feeling human beings, but it didn't work. The culture is different. Never mind. Their advice is concise, well written and immensely useful. You will find that you have bought two excellent and complementary books for the price of one.

USING CBT IN GENERAL PRACTICE by Lee David (2006)

Talking of consciousness, how much do you know about cognitive–behavioural therapy (CBT)? It seems to offer an effective approach to psychological problems within a realistic time frame, and it is supported by an impressive amount of evidence. But very few of my patients have ever had any because it is so difficult to access in the NHS at present. The next question is 'Can I learn to do it myself? And is it possible to use CBT ideas in an ordinary 10-minute consultation?'

Dr Lee David believes that it is. She is a GP who also works part-time as a trained CBT therapist, and she has written a book called *Using CBT in General Practice*. However, don't be nervous. Lee does not advise trying to do full-scale therapy during your morning surgery. Her suggestion is that GP readers could learn some of the basic principles and then use what she calls the 'cognitive–behavioural model' to help a variety of patients to manage their symptoms and their lives. The basic idea underpinning the CBM is that thoughts, feelings, behaviour and physical symptoms all affect one another in a circular way. Thus a disturbing negative thought such as 'Nobody likes me' might lead to feelings of depression, a withdrawal from social activity and the physical symptom of being tired all the time. Dr David shows how we can invite a patient to collaborate with the doctor in a process of 'guided discovery.' Together they can identify (and write down) the different components and the way that they influence each other. Hopefully this will enable the patient to understand what is going on when a minor adverse event plunges him into despair; and will equip him to deal with it more effectively. The book is a very practical learning manual. Each chapter contains theoretical sections, case studies, exercises, summaries and helpful diagrams. There is an excellent chapter on 'heart-sink' patients which shows you how to use the method on yourself and develop a more positive attitude to the patients whom you dread. This section is not so different from Balint – just a bit more cognitive. The book concludes with a series of chapters that apply the CBM to a variety of clinical problems, including depression, health anxiety and chronic physical illness. You should definitely read this book. Your registrar will want to borrow it, so take a copy for her as well.

OPENING SKINNER'S BOX: GREAT PSYCHOLOGICAL EXPERIMENTS OF THE TWENTIETH CENTURY by Lauren Slater (2004)

Next, I'd like to show an amazing collection of true stories. It's by Lauren Slater, an American psychiatrist and writer whose dreamy and rather attractive face looks out at us from inside the back cover. For this book Lauren has investigated the life and work of a string of legendary psychologists. Their experiments were simple, perhaps even crude and naive, but they all make us think 'Just what the hell sort of people are we?' She starts with BF Skinner, the founder of behaviourism. In the 1930s he built some special boxes for his rats and taught them to obtain food pellets by pressing a lever. Soon they were eagerly pressing away, even if it took three or even ten attempts to obtain their reward. More worryingly, if the food only arrived occasionally and at random intervals, the rats would still go on pressing the lever hopefully, and this behaviour was the hardest to eradicate. Remind you of anyone? Lauren points out that we humans are not much brighter than Skinner's rats. Think of the fruit machine gamblers at Las Vegas and, even more poignantly, of the girl who keeps returning to a violent man in the hope that this time he will show her some kindness. When will we ever learn?

The next case history is that of Stanley Milgram in the 1950s. He conducted the notorious experiments in which volunteer students from Yale were easily persuaded to give what they imagined were painful, even lethal electric shocks to other 'subjects', who were really actors who were only pretending to scream. Milgram found to his surprise that 65% of the students were quite willing to administer the 'torture' if they were firmly reminded that it was necessary to complete the experiment. Just obeying orders, you see. You won't need to be reminded of those other young Americans happily abusing prisoners in Baghdad. There are ten experimental psychology classics in the book, but I only have space to tell you about one more. I have chosen the work of Dr David Rosenhan, who arranged for eight sane volunteers (including himself) to present themselves for treatment at American psychiatric hospitals. They all said that they were hearing voices and that the voices said 'Thud.' That was all. They were compulsorily admitted to the wards for 'many days', given medication (which they didn't take, but neither did most of the 'real' patients), and finally released with a diagnosis of 'paranoid schizophrenia.' Of course it wouldn't happen today. Or would it? Our intrepid author decided to repeat the experiment in the twenty-first century. She, too, was given a diagnosis of 'psychosis' and was offered risperidone. The big difference was that she wasn't admitted and she was treated with great consideration and kindness. It's so good to know that psychiatry has made some progress. This is a great book that will make you chuckle, shudder, gasp and wonder.

CONSCIOUSNESS RECONNECTED: MISSING LINKS BETWEEN SELF, NEUROSCIENCE, PSYCHOLOGY AND THE ARTS by Derek Steinberg (2006)

Every now and then I suddenly catch myself wondering who on earth I am and what I'm doing here. Who is this person who is me? And why am I constantly monitoring everything around me and engaging in apparently purposeful activities? I snap out of it after a few seconds to avoid madness, but what is happening in those few seconds of detachment is that I am trying to understand what it means to be conscious. Derek Steinberg is a psychiatrist who has been puzzling over the subject for a long time and has now presented his provisional conclusions in this marvellous book called *Consciousness Reconnected*, which I urge you all to read. So what is consciousness? Well, it's the quality of being aware of yourself as 'I', a person, and also of the world around you. You almost certainly need a cerebral cortex to do consciousness and know who you are (or to know who you *think* you are) but, says Derek, neuroscience is not enough. In his wide-ranging exploration he draws ideas and evidence from philosophy, psychoanalysis, attachment theory, Jungian archetypes, evolutionary biology, artistic creation, culture and theology. He uses metaphors to help us to get a clearer sighting of our elusive quarry. Consciousness is like a film or a circus or a carousel. It's all a kind of wonderful illusion. But how can we understand what it is and where it came from when we are using our own consciousness as the instrument to dissect it? I have to admit that I found it difficult to follow some of the arguments of the more abstruse thinkers quoted by Derek, but I never felt lost for long. The author's onward drive and exhilaration carried me along until the wonderful Chapter Nine, in which he puts everything together and sums it up in a diagram rather like a Catherine wheel. Of course it's only an approximation, but I really felt that I had at least a rough idea of how we started as a single-celled amoeba that was 'aware' of good and bad things in the primeval soup, and worked our way to being a person with dreams, memories and opinions. Congratulations to Derek on a brilliant, intellectually challenging piece of work and an enjoyable read.

RUSSIAN THINKERS by Isaiah Berlin (1978)

A couple of years ago, I went to the National Theatre to see Tom Stoppard's trilogy *The Coast of Utopia*, which is all about the lives of the nineteenth-century Russian Socialists. Of course I knew about Marx (who makes a brief appearance), but I had never come across characters such as Vissarion Belinsky, Mikhail Bakunin and Alexander Herzen. Herzen is Stoppard's hero because, unlike his more violent and impulsive friends, he believed that personal liberty was more important than theory. He couldn't see the sense of having a violent revolution in which thousands would die in the hope that the next generation would construct a perfect society.

During one of the intervals I browsed at the bookstall and came across a book called *Russian Thinkers*, a collection of essays by Isaiah Berlin. This is my chance, I thought, to learn more about Herzen and his comrades and to introduce a bit of political philosophy to the Green Bookshop's shelves. I am aware that, unlike my distinguished and erudite predecessors, I have not offered my readers any books by Deep Thinkers (or, as Hyman Kaplan would call them, Dip Tinkers). Sir Isaiah provides sparkling accounts of the lives and works of all the main characters in Stoppard's plays (Stoppard must have written his script with *Russian Thinkers* at his elbow). But the chapter I enjoyed most was the first one – Berlin's celebrated essay called 'The Hedgehog and the Fox.'

He starts with a quotation from the ancient Greek poet Archilocus: 'The fox knows many things but the hedgehog knows one big thing.' Berlin then uses this comparison as a metaphor, and suggests that all writers and thinkers (and perhaps all people) are basically either foxes or hedgehogs. The hedgehogs are those who 'relate everything to a single central vision' – a grand theory which they use to underpin their lives. It might be their religion or their political beliefs, or it might be evidence-based medicine or clinical governance or the latest managerial system. The foxes, on the other hand, see a world that is full of confusing details and individual differences – no two people and no two situations are the same, and you have to pursue all sorts of different aims, some of them contradictory, and be very adaptable to circumstances. So, for example, Plato, Hegel and Marx are hedgehogs, while Aristotle and other philosophers who go more for the differences and the details are of the foxy persuasion. Dante with his firmly constructed moral universe is a hedgehog, while Shakespeare, for whom there are fewer certainties, is a fox.

But when Sir Isaiah comes to consider Tolstoy, he finds it hard to put him in either category. Here is a novelist who is a brilliant observer of the disorganised detail of human life – surely he ought to be a fox. But Tolstoy is also desperate to find a really good overall theory of history. In *War and Peace* he rubbishes all the existing historians who have attempted to explain why great events happen, but he can't really find anything convincing to put in their place. And what really is the meaning of life? He thinks he knows, but it's hard to explain. The best place to find it seems to be in a simple, natural relationship with your family and with nature, as enjoyed by the (idealised) Russian peasant. But trying to perfect and articulate this vision seems to drive him crazy. The poor chap is a natural fox who longs to be a hedgehog. As I finished the essay it occurred to me that family doctors are natural foxes, too. Every patient is a different person with a different problem, there are no rules, there are hardly any solutions, mostly you just have to listen, and grand theories are of little practical help. And yet the hedgehogs will come

CHAPTER 15

Reading for pleasure

I hope you have enjoyed your visits to the Green Bookshop and taken away plenty of books with you. There is really nothing so good as a book to have as a companion when you are bored, lonely, seeking stimulation, on a long journey, trying to find the answer to something or looking to explore pastures new.

How do you find time for reading?

When people ask me how I find time for all this reading, I don't know what sort of answer they expect. I might say, how do you find time for eating or watching football or jogging round the park? How do you find time for relationships or going to the pub? The answer is that we all have time for the things we value most and that we couldn't bear to do without. For me, reading is pretty high on the list of essential activities, so the question of finding time for it doesn't arise. That doesn't mean I am able to read everything I want to read. There are just too many books trying to tempt me to open their pages and get involved. I'm afraid I'm not very faithful to the book I promised to read first. If another one comes along and gives me the eye, I will probably fall for it and start reading that one, too. Even with two books I am tempted to stray because books are so irresistible. So I usually have not less than six books on the go at any one time. Some I will be halfway through, while I will only have read a few pages of others before I decide that they will have to wait, because good and worthy as they are, something much more sexy has come along and I have to read that first. Sometimes a book will get fed up with waiting and just lose itself among all the other books in the Bookshop (not to mention all those at home). On the other hand, there are some books that I get disenchanted with quite quickly and just give up on. The prose seems too tortuous, the sentences too long, the country I am travelling through is too rough and prickly. I do not feel guilty about this at all, because if the book is a good one, sooner or later I will pick it up again and this time the difficulties may have gone. The thorn bushes that blocked my path will have disappeared and I can romp over springy grassland with wonderful views of the surrounding hills until I reach the end. It may be months or even years before this happens. The reason is probably that there has been a change in me and I am now ready for the book in a way that I wasn't before. Does this happen to you? I hope so, because it's a very joyous experience and it shows you that you need never feel bad about not being able to read a book that everyone says is wonderful. You may just not be ready for it.

'Literary' novels

You have probably noticed that the Green Bookshop stocks only so-called 'literary' novels. These are the ones by rather highbrow authors that tend to win or be short-listed for prestigious prizes, whereas there are other novels that you won't see on our shelves that sell millions of copies and give pleasure to lots of people. Is this snobbery or what? You deserve an explanation. The fact is that we seriously prefer the literary novels because, although the best-sellers may tell a terrific story and are easy to read, a good literary novel will deliver something extra. And just what is the extra ingredient?

Well, it's not really an ingredient. It's more the texture and flavour of the whole thing. It's hard to grasp and explain just what that special quality is, but I will do my best. And if you are not convinced, I shall not mind (well, not too much), because there is a good case for saying it's all a matter of taste and what sort of book happens to appeal to you. There is no way I can prove that literary novels are 'better.' I can only tell you what they do for me.

I am thinking of modern authors such as Ian McEwan, Philip Roth, Salman Rushdie, Sebastian Faulks, AL Kennedy and Kazuo Ishiguro, all of whom you will have seen on our shelves. And of course the classics, but I'll come to them later. These authors and many others have a special ability to use language in a way that sets up all sorts of pleasurable responses in me. Their descriptions stir up a variety of sensory impressions – sights, sounds, smells and touches – that make me feel as if I am actually experiencing the world they are describing. Their language can be poetic, moving, disturbing and also very humorous and entertaining. They can use irony to add an extra layer to a character's point of view. They can create characters who are complicated and ambiguous, just like real people. These characters can remind me of aspects of myself. Some writers (such as George Eliot or Henry James) can give a very detailed account of a character's state of mind. Others use the 'stream of consciousness' narrative, which makes you feel as if you are inside a person's head. And despite the importance of subjectivity, there is also pleasure in watching the writer at work, seeing from a slightly detached position just how cleverly she does it. And when we come to the classic writers (Tolstoy, Jane Austen, Dickens, and so on), they just did all these things so well that their books are still enjoyed many years after the authors are gone. You can read them over and over again and always get pleasure and always find something new. And there I rest my case.

Before or after?

We hope that our reviews will have given you a keen desire to get hold of some of the books we have so lovingly described, and to read them for yourselves. If you belong to a book club, you may have got some ideas for your next choice. Dorothy is always telling me about her book club, and I'd love to join, but apparently it's for women only.

That's not strictly true, we did have a man once but he was disruptive. And at the moment we are full, but I'll let you know if there's a vacancy. Thanks, Dorothy. I'd be very well behaved. I'm just so curious about what you girls get up to. *I doubt if it's as exciting as you think. But it can be very enjoyable to talk or read about a book you already know, and see what other people think.* Exactly. And I hope you will also have enjoyed agreeing or disagreeing with what we have to say about the books you have already read.

What about the medical books if you are not a doctor?

Yes, it will be clear by now that the Green Bookshop was created with doctors, and especially GPs, in mind. We wanted to supply them with lots of good novels and a sprinkling of non-medical non-fiction to give them a break from their work and also to broaden and stimulate their minds. But we also showcase (if I may use the word) the best books we can find that shed light on general practice. Now if you are not a GP or a primary healthcare worker you may think that this part of the Green Bookshop holds nothing for you. This is emphatically not the case! Our medical books are not very technical because general practice is an art as well as a science and is essentially about people. Most of our medical books are very accessible to the non-medical reader, and we hope that they will be of interest. We have books about the present state of the NHS and the way it is likely to develop (not altogether reassuring). As a user of the NHS this is important for you to know about! We also show you how doctors are being educated in the twenty-first century and how they struggle with the art of the consultation, which is where doctor and patient meet and try to understand one another. Finally, we have a number of books about our states of mind and what exactly we mean by such labels as 'depression', which is compelling reading for everyone. So if you have walked past the Medical Section of our store, we urge you to pop back and take another look.

Finally

Dorothy and I have so much enjoyed these sessions with you. *And we hope that you have, too.* Enjoy your reading, and don't forget to call again soon!

Index of authors: fiction and non-fiction

Index of authors:
medical titles

Index of fiction titles

Index of non-fiction titles

Index of medical titles

Arts in Medical Education, The by Elaine Powley and Roger Higson (Radcliffe Publishing, 2005) **127–8**

Bandolier's Little Book of Making Sense of the Medical Evidence by Andrew Moore and Henry McQuay (Oxford University Press, 2006) **112–13**

Behind the Consultation by André Matalon and Stanley Rabin (Radcliffe Publishing, 2007) **118**

Beyond Depression: a new approach to understanding and management by Christopher Dowrick (Oxford University Press, 2004) **129–31**

Challenge for Primary Care, The by Nigel Starey (Radcliffe Medical Press, 2003) **109–10**

Cinemeducation: a Comprehensive Guide to Using Film in Medical Education edited by Matthew Alexander, Patricia Lenahan and Ann Pavlov (Radcliffe Publishing, 2005) **74–5**

Communication Skills That Heal by Barry Bub (Radcliffe Publishing, 2006) **115–16**

Condensed Curriculum Guide, The: for GP training and the MCGP by Ben Riley, Jayne Haynes and Steve Field (RCGP, 2008) **124–5**

Complexity in Primary Care: understanding its value by Kieran Sweeney (Radcliffe Medical Press, 2006) **106–7**

Consciousness Reconnected by Derek Steinberg (Radcliffe Publishing, 2006) **135–6**

Differential Diagnosis in Dermatology by Richard Ashton and Barbara Leppard (Radcliffe Publishing, 2004) **114**

Doctor, His Patient and the Illness, The by Michael Balint (1957) Millennium edition (Churchill Livingstone, 2000) (currently out of print) **95–6**

Doctors Talking to Patients (1976) by Patrick Byrne and Barrie Long (RCGP, 1984) **96–8**

From General Practice to Primary Care: the industrialisation of family medicine by Steve Iliffe (Oxford University Press, 2008) **107–9**

Fortunate Man, A by John Berger and Jean Mohr (1969) (RCGP Publications, 2003) **98–100, 112**

Inner Consultation, The by Roger Neighbour (1987) (Radcliffe Publishing, 2005) **102–3**

Listening as Work in Primary Care by Simon Cocksedge (Radcliffe Publishing, 2005) **116–17**

Matters of Life and Death: key writings by Iona Heath (Radcliffe Publishing, 2008) **110–12**